David Ip

Casebook of Orthopedic Rehabilitation

David Ip

Casebook of Orthopedic Rehabilitation

Including Virtual Reality

With 74 Figures and 1 Table

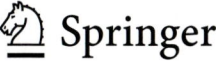 Springer

Dr. David Ip
MBBS (HKU), FRCS (Ed) Orth, FHKCOS,
FHKAM (Orthopedic Surg), FIBA (UK), FABI (USA)
Deputy Governor,
American Biographical Institute Research Association (USA)
Hon Director General (Asia)
of International Biographical Association of Cambridge (UK)

ISBN 978-3-540-74426-9   e-ISBN 978-3-540-74427-6

DOI 10.1007/978-3-540-74427-6

Library of Congress Control Number: 2007933703

© 2008 Springer-Verlag Berlin Heidelberg

Cover design: Frido Steinen-Broo, eStudio Calamar, Spain

Printed on acid-free paper
9 8 7 6 5 4 3 2 1

springer.com

About the Author

Dr. David Ip is a fellow of various professional organizations, including the Royal College of Surgeons and the Hong Kong College of Orthopedic Surgeons, and is a member of the American Academy of Orthopedic Surgeons and the American Association of Academic Physiatrists, among many others, such as the International Association for the Study of Pain and various Gait Analysis societies. His biography is included in *Marquis Who's Who in Science & Engineering, Who's Who in Medicine and Healthcare, Sterling's Who's Who in NY*, and the *International Who's Who Historical Society*. In his capacity as Director General (Asia) of the International Biographical Association of the UK and as Clinical Governor of the American Biographical Institute he has contributed significantly to peer-reviewed journal articles and has written several books on orthopedics, which have received positive reviews from the Royal College of Surgeons and the *Journal of Bone and Joint Surgery*. He is also the reviewer of selected orthopedic journals published in Europe, and holds honorary consultancy positions for various companies like the Lehrman Gerson group, Brand's Institute, Medacorp, among many others.

Preface

As the name implies, this "casebook" contains a series of clinical cases on various topics in orthopedic rehabilitation that the author encountered over his 23 years of practice ranging from the extremely common conditions like knee arthritis, to newer technologies evolved in the recent years including the use of smart materials in orthopedics, hypergravity stimulation therapy, and virtual reality.

Many of us must have encountered difficult real life hurdles to rehabilitation in real clinical practice in which patients have difficulty in coming back for rehabilitation either because they live very far away, or they do not really have adequate time, or they simply only agree for home-based rehabilitation for various reasons. In these case scenarios, no matter how good a "protocol" one has on hand, it will be difficult to achieve the expected result. When the author was still young, he made the common mistake of accepting lesser outcomes from these patients saying to myself that it is a question of compliance. However, with large strides in computer engineering, even rural district patients can have acceptable rehabilitation as long as they have a telephone line and the right computer hardware and software and input-output devices to effect tele-rehabilitation via the aid of virtual reality rather than just relying on video conferencing alone.

Although this book is a close companion of its fellow, "Orthopedic Rehabilitation, Assessment, and Enablement" which is very well received in many parts of the world, it can however be used alone as all the clinical cases stand alone and are self-contained. Each case scenario is based on real clinical situation (except the one on space travel*) seen by the author during his clinical practice or during his visits to overseas centers although the names and some fine details of patients were changed to protect their privacy. Finally, a wide readership is expected of this book including primary care physicians, fellow orthopedic surgeons, physiatrists, therapists, orthopedic nurses and senior medical students. Happy Reading!

David Ip
Hong Kong, October 2007

---

* To enhance protection of privacy of SARS patients, the MRI Knee of Case number 28 was selected from a Non-SARS patient but with extremely similar pattern of involvement as the original patient

Contents

Section II

SECTION I

**Case Illustrations
of the Rehabilitation
of Common and Challenging
Orthopedic Conditions**

New Dual-energy X-ray Absorptiometry Machines (iDXA) and Vertebral Fracture Assessment (VFA)

History and Examination

Your wealthy friend who is a banker brings his 62-year-old mother to your office one day with worries concerning his mother Jenny's progressive height loss over the past year. Her recent dual-energy X-ray absorptiometry (DXA) report showed a T-score of –2.0 and on and off dull back aches. Jenny has no history of previously documented fragility fractures, no maternal history of such fractures, and no chronic use of drugs. Your banker friend has consulted two clinicians before consulting you: One suggested prophylactic bisphosphonates based on the DXA report, and the other suggested only a high calcium diet, paying attention to life-style factors like adequate exercise and sunshine, with no need for treatment.

After educating your banker friend that nowadays our tendency to treat osteoporosis relies more on risk calculation rather than on a number known as the T-score, you refer Jenny to have the new vertebral fracture (VFA) assessment after noting local tenderness at the thoracolumbar junction and around the L4 vertebra, as well as somewhere near the mid-thoracic spine.

Your banker friend agrees to the arrangement and is pleased to note that the amount of radiation dose will be significantly lower than that of conventional radiographs. The VFA was performed by a new center that is equipped with a state-of-the-art high-resolution new iDXA machine, and the report shows grade 2 vertebral collapse on the Genant scale at T7, T12 and L4 multiple vertebral levels. Based on these important new findings, you decide to treat Jenny with a combination of calcium, and the newer weekly bisphosphonates (that has incorporated vitamin D inside the tablets), as well as referring her to the physical therapists for postural training and lumbar stabilization exercise. Describe how the newer popular VFA assessments can be of help in these common case scenarios seen almost daily in our orthopedic clinics.

Discussion

This case scenario illustrates clearly the current worldwide tendency to refrain from relying too heavily on a mere number known as the T-score (named after a researcher whose name begins with the letter "T"), but rather concentrate on the calculation of the risk profile of the individual of suffering from fragility fractures. In fact, the WHO is fully aware of this modern trend and has just published revised guidelines for the management of osteoporosis, not just based on a number (T-score), but with stresses on risk calculation and assessment (Iki, Clin Calcium, 2007).

Some of us may ask why we should rely on risk calculation rather than a number (or bone mass) to which we have grown accustomed. This is because if one refers to the definition of osteoporosis, we notice that these individuals have *concomitant* deterioration in bone architecture, not just loss in bone mass. Thus, some patients with documented fragility fractures after very low energy injury to their skeleton do not have a T-score of –2.5 or lower; in these individuals, it is believed that the significant deterioration in the bony micro-architecture is at work here, and this definitely warrants treatment. For these cases, it is the bony architecture or quality that is mainly at fault.

Disadvantage of Conventional X-ray in Assessing the Presence of Vertebral Fractures in the Thoracic and Lumbar Spine

Even conventional radiographs of the thoracic and lumbar spines long films can be subject to diminished quality owing to different soft tissue envelope thickness, the X-ray angle of the radiographic machine, and the dose of radiation is also much higher than VFA by 15–20 times: 600 μSv vs. 30 μSv (teachings of ISCD Course 2007).

Advantages of Using VFA Instead of Conventional X-ray

Advantages include no parallax error, dual energy imaging equalizes the soft tissue variations mentioned above, and the analysis can be semi-quantitative using the guidelines of Genant reported previously in J Bone Miner Res. Most importantly, with the advent of newer high resolution DXA can reflect on morphometry, and the accuracy of detecting both clinical as well as silent thoraco-lumbar fractures will increase. Besides, there is the added advantage of much less radiation, which appeals to many patients including Jenny in the current case scenario.

The Term Vertebral Fracture Assessment

Vertebral fracture assessment (VFA) is the correct term that should be used to denote densitometric spine imaging performed for the purpose of detecting vertebral fractures.

Indication for VFA (According to ISCD Position Statement)

When BMD measurement is indicated, performance of VFA should be considered in clinical situations that may be associated with vertebral fractures (as determined by the attending clinician).

Common examples include:

- Documented height loss of greater than 2 cm (0.75 in) or historical height loss greater than 4 cm (1.5 in) since young adulthood
- History of fracture after age 50
- Commitment to long-term oral or parenteral glucocorticoid therapy
- History and/or findings suggestive of vertebral fracture not documented by prior radiologic study

Pitfalls

- The methodology utilized for vertebral fracture identification should be similar to standard radiological approaches and be provided in the report.
- Fracture diagnosis should be based on visual evaluation and include assessment of grade/severity. Morphometry *alone* is not recommended because it is unreliable for diagnosis.

- The severity of vertebral fractures may be determined using the semi-quantitative assessment criteria developed by Genant (J Bone Miner Res, 1993). Severity of the deformity may be confirmed by morphometric measurement if desired.
- For example, additional imaging can be considered when there are equivocal fractures, unidentifiable vertebrae between T7 and L4, sclerotic or lytic changes, or findings suggestive of conditions other than osteoporosis. VFA is designed to detect vertebral fracture and not other abnormalities.

Newer High-resolution DXA Machines

One high-resolution DXA machine that is ideal for assessing VFA is the iDXA, a product by GE Healthcare. According to GE, iDXA (Fig. 1) can produce sharper images and with the best precision and accuracy. It was FDA-approved in 2005.

Main features of iDXA include:

- Improved precision in the measurement of the bone that is brought about by the CZT-HD detector, allowing clinicians to track changes previously too minor to detect, faster than before. This allows physicians to better manage osteoporosis treatment plans by offering feedback faster.
- The six-point calibration technique eases assessment of vertebral shape and morphology (Fig. 2).
- Besides the capability of non-invasive measurement of skeletal bone status, the new product can also measure lean and fat tissue components including percentage fat, lean tissue mass.

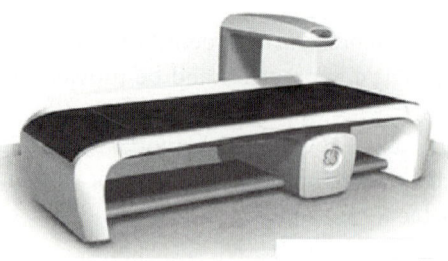

Fig. 1 The iDXA machine, an example of a newer generation of DXA machine (courtesy of General Electric)

Biomechanics of Height Loss in Elders

The biomechanics of age-related spinal deformity of vertebral bone loss and disc degeneration associated with aging causes bone and disc structures to weaken and deform as a result of gravity and postural stresses.

Recently, an anatomically accurate sagittal-plane, upright-posture biomechanical model of the anterior spinal column (C2–S1) was created by digitizing lateral full-spine radiographs of 20 human subjects with a mean height of 176.8 cm and a mean body weight of 76.6 kg. Body weight loads were applied to the model, after which intervertebral disc and vertebral body forces and deformation were computed and the new spine geometry was calculated. The strength and stiffness of the vertebral bodies were reduced according to an osteopenic aging model and modulus reduction algorithm respectively.

It was found that the most osteopenic model produced gross deformities of the spine, including anterior wedge-like fracture deformities at T7 and T8. In this model, increases in thoracic kyphosis and decreases in vertebral body height resulted in a 25% decrease in spinal height (C2–S1), an 8% decrease in total body height, and a 15.1-cm anterior translation of the C2 spine segment centroid. The resulting deformity qualitatively resembled deformities observed in elderly individuals with osteoporotic compression fractures.

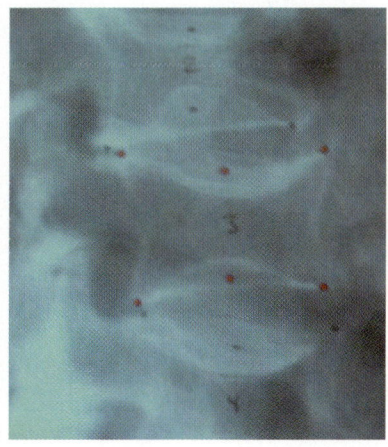

Fig. 2 Six-point calibration method

The findings suggest that postural forces are responsible for the initiation of osteoporotic spinal deformity in elderly subjects. Vertebral deformities are exacerbated by anterior translation of the upper spinal column, which increases compressive loads in the thoraco-lumbar region of the spine (Keller et al., Spine, 2003).

However, it was pointed out in other recent studies that height loss in the elderly is *not* invariably due to osteoporotic vertebral collapse at one or more level and that there are other possibilities. But owing to the disadvantages of conventional radiographs in screening the whole spine, the new high-resolution DXA machine such as iDXA from GE will prove to be a very useful screening tool and will help the orthopedic surgeon in determining the status of the vertebral column as well as aid in the decision-making process concerning the management of osteoporosis.

Present Case Scenario

Jenny was found to have multiple levels of relatively silent vertebral collapse, coupled age and T-score considerations; you started Jenny on bisphosphonates therapy.

Learning Point

The use of VFA is expected to increase in the coming years for several reasons:

- The paradigm shift in measuring absolute fracture risk besides treating a number (bone mass) as in the past.
- Newer high resolution DXA mentioned provides the needed resolution for detecting vertebral collapse fracture over the whole thoraco-lumbar region and help in many cases the decision-making process of whether to start as well as how to give anti-osteoporosis treatment.
- Much less radiation and the same machine investigates not only bone mass but vertebral details of the whole spine.

References

1. Keller TS, Harrison DE, et al. (2003) Prediction of osteoporotic spinal deformity. Spine, 28(5):455–62
2. Iki M (2007) Absolute risk for fracture and WHO guideline: WHO model for assessing absolute risk of fractures. Clin Calcium 17:7, 1015–21

History and Examination

Jennifer is a 79-year-old retired secretary. She has a history of recurrent falls and fractured her left distal radius 2 years ago, followed by left hip pertrochanteric fracture treated by a dynamic hip screw last year by your orthopedic unit. Jennifer's mother had also had a fragility hip fracture in the past 1 year before she passed away due to a cardiovascular event. This admission, Jennifer presents with back pain and a radiograph reveals a wedge compression vertebral fracture at the L1 vertebra after minor trauma. She had a DXA scan done last year with a T-score of –2.6. All along she has refused medication for osteoporosis, including bisphosphonates, calcium/vitamin D, etc., as she finds it very tedious taking the pills. She remembers being given some calcium and vitamin D tablets after her initial fragility fracture 2 years ago, but another doctor stopped these pills in a subsequent follow-up and Jennifer thought these pills were therefore not essential for her health. Moreover, as she felt there was decreased pain at her left wrist, there was no point in taking these medications. She also heard that one of her friends developed an esophageal ulcer after taking bisphosphonates and she is not particularly keen to have this drug either. In view of three fragility fractures in a row, how will you proceed to manage this lady with osteoporosis and fall risks, yet who refuses any kind of oral drugs?

Discussion

Not infrequently, clinicians dealing with patients with fragility fractures may encounter patients who refuse to take all kinds of medications. One way of helping to maintain bone mass, and at the same time recruit Type 2 muscle fiber in fall prevention for this group of elderly involves "hyper-gravity stimulation," sometimes also called "vibration therapy." This method of training was first started by Russian scientists due to their desire to keep astronauts in better physical condition during space travel.

Nature of Hyper-gravity Stimulation Training

Essentially a neuromuscular training method using low to moderate vertical vibration stimulus to improve muscle strength and power. Effects depend on amplitude, frequency, duration, and positioning of the patient on the machine. There are two types of such machines: "Pivoting type" vs. the "linear type."

- Pivot-type machine:
  - Advantages: This design is based on the normal human walking pattern, thus evoking both vertical and horizontal balance reflexes (Fig. 3).
  - Disadvantages: Stimulant effect limited to below the pelvic line, only about 10 different training positions can be performed, and cannot adjust amplitude with the same position, rather noisy with higher frequency, sometimes may even cause nausea at high frequency.

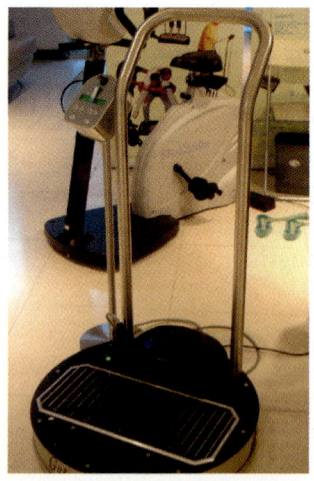

Fig. 3 Popular hyper-gravity stimulation machine under the brand name Galileo

- Linear-type machines:
  - Advantages: The most effective mechanism to accelerate gravity force, many more positioning possibilities, and can control amplitude without changing the patient's position.

Selection of Machine Type

In general, stainless steel materials transmit forces best; with an increase in platform size, there are more possibilities of having different training positions. The setting of training frequency range should not be < 20 Hz since too low a frequency can cause resonance of internal organs. Commonly used frequencies range between 20 and 45 Hz, while the amplitude range is from 1 to 5 mm. The duration of training per session is about 5–15 min, starting from 5 min in the elderly and slowly increasing as the patient's tolerance improves. The position of training varies depending on which muscle group the therapist wishes to train, and the efficiency of training is improved in the presence of preliminary stretched muscle. A machine of adequate weight is needed since the forces of acceleration can reach as high as 10 G in some cases.

Mechanism of Action

It is believed that hyper-gravity stimulation works by the following mechanism:

- Gravity acceleration: Degree of acceleration is the product of amplitude and frequency. The hyper-stimulation method elicits loading to the musculoskeletal system by an increase in gravitational loading.
- Tonic vibration reflex: Continuous small stretch on muscles by vertical vibration. Muscle spindles notice this change and pass it on to the spinal cord, to effect reflex contraction of the stimulated muscle groups. In effect, vibration therapy enhances excitatory inflow from muscle spindles to the motor neuron pools and depresses the inhibitory impact of the Golgi Tendon Organ due to the accommodation of vibration stimuli.

Possible Benefits of Hyper-gravity Training

- Increases muscle strength and power not only in young untrained individuals (Roelants et al., Int J Sports Med, 2004), but even in the elderly (Roelants et al., J Am Geriatr Soc, 2004).
- Increases bone density (Verschueren et al., J Bone Miner Res, 2004).
- Improves co-ordination and proprioception and postural control, even in elderly (Verschueren et al., J Bone Miner Res, 2004).
- Improves flexibility and recruits previously inactive muscle fibers.
- Activates and recruits Type II muscle fibers in the elderly, and relieves muscle tension and joint adhesions. In one study in older adults: In ladies aged 58–74 over a 24-week period, isometric and dynamic knee extensor strength increased significantly in the vibration group, as did speed of knee movement (J Sports Sci, 2006).
- Increases explosive strength in athletes (Issurin et al., J Sports Sci, 1999). In sport, mechanical vibration is used as a massage tool and/ or for training purposes. Two varieties of vibration training can be distinguished: Strength exercises with superimposed vibratory stimulation (VS) and motor tasks performed under whole body vibration (WBV; Issurin et al., J Sports Med Phys Fitness, 2005). In comparison to VS exercises, WBV tasks generate more global neuromuscular, metabolic and hormonal responses. Whole body vibration training resulted in significant changes in several motor variables, with stretch-shortening cycle tests (such as countermovement jumps, serial high jumps, etc.) being the most sensitive to whole body vibration treatment.

Present Case Scenario

Jennifer agreed to undergo hypergravity stimulation therapy, and tolerated it well. She had a total of four courses, each interposed 3 months apart. After the training, Jennifer claimed a subjective increase in general well-being, more confidence in walking and going out on her own, and performs IADL activities adequately.

Learning Point

- Hyper-gravity stimulation therapy or vibration therapy works by gravity acceleration and stimulation of tonic vibration reflex.

- Suitable administration of vibration therapy not only helps to build up muscle strength and power in the elderly, but also increases bone density in these individuals. It is the author's view that this therapy can be offered to patients who refuse drug treatment for osteoporosis, or used as an adjunct to those who do agree to take medication. There is also added evidence to show that the therapy may improve co-ordination and proprioception and postural control in the elderly and possibly prevent falls and related injuries in this patient population.

- The current case scenario describes a patient who refuses osteoporosis medications; for those patients who agree to take osteoporosis medications, one should refer to the latest WHO guidelines (Gorai, Clin Calcium, 2007).

References

1. Roelants M, Delecluse C, et al. (2004) Whole-body-vibration training increases knee extension strength and speed of movement in older women. J Am Geriatr Soc, 52(6):901–8

2. Roelants M, Delecluse C, et al. (2004) Effects of 24 weeks of whole body vibration training on body composition and muscle strength in untrained females. Int J Sports Med, 25(1):1–5

3. Verschueren SM, Roelants M, et al. (2004) Effect of 6-month whole body vibration training on hip density, muscle strength, and postural control in postmenopausal women: a randomized controlled pilot study. J Bone Miner Res, 19(3):352–9

4. Issurin VB, Tenenbaum G, et al. (1999) Acute and residual effects of vibratory stimulation on explosive strength in elite and amateur athletes. J Sports Sci, 17(3):177–82

5. Issurin VB (2005) Vibrations and their applications in sport. A review. J Sports Med Phys Fitness, 45(3):324–36

6. Gorai I (2007) Absolute risk of fracture and WHO Guideline: Selection of drugs for the prevention of fractures in postmenopausal women. Clin Calcium, 17:7,1090–6

Lady Having Difficulty in Controlling the Computer Mouse

History and Examination

Veronica is a 29-year-old right-handed computer graphics designer. She first presented to her family physician with complaints of "difficulty in performing the right and left mouse clicks" while executing Corel Draw software using her right hand. Then she noticed difficulty in maneuvering the whole mouse, which always tended to drift to one side.

The family doctor referred Veronica to you to "rule out" any orthopedic problems. You examined Veronica, but the upper limb neurological examination was normal apart from mild apparent weakness in the right hand FHL and index finger FDP function. Examination of the sensory system including 2-point discrimination was normal as was examination of the cervical spine. Bilateral Phalen's and Tinel's signs were negative. There were no clinical signs to suggest thoracic outlet syndrome.

You ordered radiological assessment of the cervical spine and blood work, and arranged for Veronica to return to the clinic in 6 weeks' time.

Despite the lack of positive radiological and hematological findings, Veronica's symptoms worsened. You checked for the "O" sign on physical assessment and the findings were as shown in Fig. 4.

You subsequently arranged nerve conduction testing (Fig. 5) with results pointing to your initial suspicion of anterior interosseous nerve entrapment.

Subsequent surgical intervention contributed to slow but sure recovery of the right hand function.

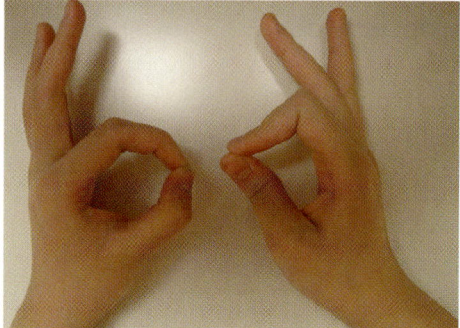

Fig. 4 Typical "O" sign seen in anterior interosseous nerve palsy

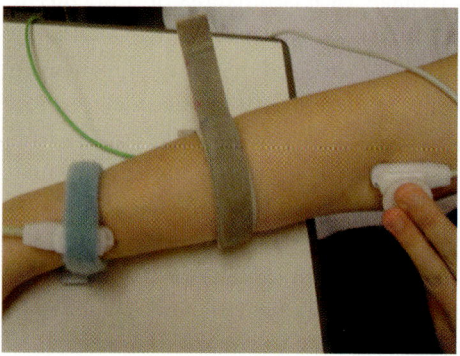

Fig. 5 Set-up for the performance of nerve conduction testing assessment checking for anterior interosseous nerve palsy by the dorsal recording method described in the text

Discussion

In Fig. 5, one can see that the patient's elbow is flexed 90° and the forearm pronated, with the stimulation electrode at elbow level at the usual site of stimulation of the median nerve; while the neutral ground electrode is in the dorsal aspect of the mid-forearm. The recording electrode is 3 cm proximal to the ulna styloid at the dorsal distal forearm with its corresponding nearby reference electrode at the ulna styloid prominence.

The author has found this method of nerve testing for anterior interosseous nerve palsy (AIN) first reported by Mysiw and Colachis (Am J Phys Med Rehabil, 1988) to be very useful, for it is non-invasive, and yet still has the advantage of recoding the effect of isolated stimulation of AIN distal to the pronator teres muscle, thus easing differentiation between neurapraxia and complete axonal loss in AIN injury or entrapment.

An alternative technique includes percutaneous stimulation of the AIN in the volar forearm, but this is also invasive and needs a very detailed knowledge of forearm anatomy and its normal variants.

Yet, other studies using surface recordings over FPL encountered difficulty in motor point placement (Phys Ther, 1977).

Dorsal recording as illustrated in this case is very much preferred since with volar surface recordings; nerve conduction from other median nerve innervated muscles can alter the response upon median nerve stimulation at the elbow – not just muscles innervated by AIN; besides, this method is non-invasive.

Pitfalls

Note that the relatively large range of normal distal latencies (of AIN) is expected stemming from the known variability of the normal anatomy of AIN, making some practical difficulties in establishing a consistent distance between the cathode and anode, as pointed out by Mysiw and Colachis (Am J Phys Med Rehabil, 1988).

Comparison between different sides (right vs. left) was therefore done keeping the *distance constant* as far as possible. Under such circumstances, a latency difference of 0.4 ms can be deemed abnormal or warrant further investigation and clinical correlation.

The author noted in his series of cases that there was a scatter in the amplitude of CMAP among participants and this similar finding was reported by Mysiw and Colachis. The observed phenomenon probably reflects differences in the muscle mass of the PQ (pronator quadratus), and tends to be higher in the dominant hand of the same individual.

The CMAP detected using the current methodology typically has an initial negative deflection followed by a bimodal shape, which might be explained by the anatomy of PQ having two heads, according to previous dissection studies by Johnson and co-workers.

Learning Point

- The presentation of AIN palsy can be very subtle, as in this lady, who only noticed a subtle difficulty in executing computer mouse clicks at initial presentation.
- The non-invasive dorsal surface recording method was found by the author to be very useful. A comparison of recordings of both sides is important. The method is non-invasive, does not involve needle electrodes and was found by the author to be welcomed by most patients.

References

1. Mysiw WJ, Colachis SC (1988) Electrophysiological study of the anterior interosseous nerve. Am J Phys Med Rehabil 67(2):50–4
2. Craft S, Currier DP, et al. (1977) Motor conduction of the anterior interosseous nerve. Phys Ther 57(10):1143–7

History and Examination

You saw a young 27-year-old office worker Sharon the other day at your orthopedic clinic. Sharon has persistent neck, shoulder and arm pain after a high speed acceleration-deceleration injury in a traffic accident 12 weeks ago, which is still causing severe neck pain and disability and she has been off work ever since the accident. Sharon complained of numbness over the bilateral upper limbs, dizziness, double vision, headaches and loss of balance and vertigo. She even has some discomfort in the temporo-mandibular joint and has lost 4 kg in weight that she ascribed to loss of appetite. Before being seen by you, Sharon was seen in the outpatient clinic of another hospital. During the past 12 weeks, Sharon had been having on and off physiotherapy sessions for her neck; the colleagues in the other hospital performed a flexion/extension view of the cervical spine as well as spine MRI, both of which were reported as being unremarkable with no disc herniations. A CT scan reported a very minor chip fracture at C6, which the attending spine surgeon agreed to observe. Lateral plain cervical spine radiograph did show a kyphotic deformity, however.

Twelve weeks after the injury, Sharon was first seen by your colleague who thought that many of Sharon's complaints were psychosomatic in origin and thought that she was just trying to get more sick leave. On examination, your colleague classified Sharon as having grade 2 Quebec Task Force classification of whiplash injury. Sharon still has residual local tenderness of the cervical spine associated with limitation of motion in all directions. When you examined Sharon during the second visit, she does have a few beats of nystagmus on examination on looking both to the right and left, and you noted some stiffness at Sharon's temporo-mandibular joint. You also noted that Sharon is anxious about not yet being able to be back at work, yet being thought of as a malingerer, and Sharon was almost on the verge of crying. Your nurse offered Sharon a glass of water and she choked while drinking, saying she had recently been having swallowing difficulties as well. Describe how you would proceed from here, and the management of Sharon's multiple symptomatology.

Discussion

Classification of Whiplash Injury

The most popular classification of whiplash injuries is that of the Quebec Task Force published in 1995 as a report that contained evidence-based recommendations regarding the treatment of these injuries, based on studies completed before 1993 and consensus-based recommendations.

Table 1 The Quebec Task Force Classification of Whiplash-related Disorders

Grade		Symptoms and Signs
I	No neck pain	No physical sign
IIA	Neck pain, stiffness	No signs
IIB	Neck pain	Positive signs ↓ ROM, tender
III	Neck pain	Positive signs, weakness/numb
IV	Neck pain with fracture +/– dislocation	

[Other possible symptoms include: hearing, visual, cognitive changes, dysphagia, headache, and temporo-manibular joint dysfunction]

Complex Symptomatology

Many of us involved in the treatment of whiplash injuries will notice that the manifestations of symptomatology are protean. These symptoms may be dismissed as being "psychosomatic" by a junior resident or trainee surgeon. These include:

- Psychological disturbances as reported by Adams et al. (Adams et al., J Occup Rehabil, 1977)

- Altered jaw-neck motor control as reported by Eriksson et al. (Arch Oral Biol, 2007). One should note that neck function is an integral part of natural jaw behavior, and that neck injury can impair jaw function and therefore disturb eating behavior.

- Sensory hypersensitivity, which can occur in up to 75% patients with the chronic disorder as reported by Jull et al. from Australia in Spine 2007, e.g., widespread mechanical and cold hyperalgesia. This can be assessed clinically by sensory and motor testing, range-of-motion testing, peak velocity, smoothness of movement (charted as the jerk index), and repositioning acuity after cervical rotation maneuver (Michael et al., Man Ther, 2006). Recent literature did reveal, however, a high individuality in the prevailing sensorimotor disturbances in an individual patient, and emphasizes the importance of developing *specific* rehabilitation programs for specific dysfunctions, and a programmed rehabilitation *tailored* to the individual patient (Man Ther, 2006).

- Vestibular rehabilitation is also important, and is an all too often overlooked aspect, even in multi-disciplinary programs in whiplash-associated disorders. Vestibular dysfunction is usually suggested by persistent dizziness, double vision and loss of balance. Proper vestibular rehabilitation for patients with whiplash-associated disorder has been shown to decrease self-perceived handicap and increase postural control (Ekvall et al., J Rehabil Med, 2006).

- Finally, subtle oculomotor dysfunctions can be present as hidden causes of disability following whiplash injury. The pathomechanics of these oculomotor dysfunctions is likely to be related to input disturbances of the cervical or vestibular afferents (Storaci et al., Eur Spine J, 2006).

Pathomechanics of Pain after Whiplash Injury

It is now believed that nerve sheath inflammation without significant axonal degeneration can result in the c-fibers (both axons in continuity and the nervi nervorum) becoming spontaneously active and mechanically sensitive. This may help to explain the painful responses when examining neural dynamics in many patients with nonspecific arm pain, as well as arm pain following whiplash injury, even when longitudinal nerve excursion (measured using ultrasound imaging), appears to be within normal ranges. These findings have implications for the clinical examination and treatment of these patient groups (Greening, Man Ther, 2006).

Charting of Outcome for Whiplash Injury Patients

- The VAS (visual analogue scale) is one of the most frequently used serial outcome charts.
- Besides the VAS, the author favors the use of measures like the Patient Specific Functional Scale, Pain Bothersomeness, the Whiplash Disability Questionnaire and the Dizziness Handicap Inventory (if dizziness is a prominent symptom) in serial assessment with regard to response to treatment and these have recently also been proven to be sensitive parameters for this chronic disorder (Stewart et al., Spine, 2007).

Management of the Current Case Scenario

Recently, some researchers have made rather negative comments; that there is "no known effective treatments for those people whose pain and disability persist beyond 3 months" (Spitzer et al., Spine, 2007).

It is the author's belief, however, that improvement in the degree of disability from whiplash-associated disorders can still occur, *unless* really very chronic, say > 6 months.

First, we prescribed exercise therapy for Sharon, because the latest findings revealed that exercise is more effective for patients with higher baseline pain and disability, just like our patient who has lots of pain (Ferrantelli et al., J Manipul Physiol Ther, 2005).

Setting-up of a Multi-disciplinary Team

One main aim of setting up a multidisciplinary team is to alter the patient's perception with strategies that specifically target disability beliefs – this is performed by the psychiatrist in the team.

Clinical biomechanics of posture rehabilitation methods – similar to the neutral zone concepts in the lumbar spine is stressed very much by the author. The efficacy of such therapies has in fact just been reported in the literature (J Manipul Physiol Ther, 2005). In this connection, this part of the treatment to Sharon involved:

- Mirror-image cervical spine adjustments
- Bio-feedback
- Exercise
- Gentle traction to reduce forward head posture and the cervical kyphosis

Sharon's abnormal head protrusion slowly resolved and cervical kyphosis returned to lordosis. Use of mirrors at home during exercise is encouraged for posture re-training.

Oculomotor dysfunction, if present, requires proper rehabilitation (Eur Spine J, 2006), but is not a prominent symptom in Sharon.

Shoulder and arm proprioception deficit, if found on examination should be dealt with (Sandlund et al., J Rehabil Med, 2006). In this case, emphasis was put on first regaining full ROM, then stressing the proprioceptive stimulation at the very end of motion ranges that help stimulate the firing of proprioceptive receptors, followed by isokinetics machine re-training for the shoulder.

The occupational therapist of our team meanwhile reinforced the importance of good posture as well as provision of ergonomic advice concerning the use of a visual-display unit.

Sensorimotor rehabilitation and serial assessment by a physiotherapist, with monitoring of therapy by graphical representation on the shoulder isokinetic machine were arranged.

Vestibular symptoms was present in this patient and were dealt with by ENT surgeons, and rehabilitation here involved exercises challenging and improving her balance function, head-eye coordination exer-

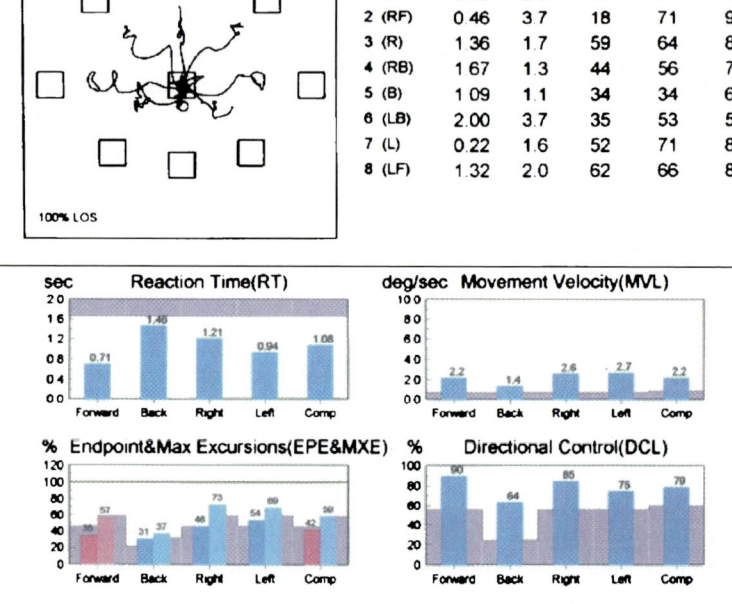

Limits Of Stability

Transition	RT (sec)	MVL (deg/sec)	EPE (%)	MXE (%)	DCL (%)
1 (F)	0.53	2.8	36	70	93
2 (RF)	0.46	3.7	18	71	90
3 (R)	1.36	1.7	59	64	88
4 (RB)	1.67	1.3	44	56	74
5 (B)	1.09	1.1	34	34	64
6 (LB)	2.00	3.7	35	53	54
7 (L)	0.22	1.6	52	71	82
8 (LF)	1.32	2.0	62	66	83

100% LOS

Data Range Note: User Data Range 70–79

Post Test Comment

Fig. 6 A typical print-out of the result of the sensory organization test, note the increased body sway even on stationary standing in this patient

cise, visual-ocular control exercise and sensory substitution-promoting exercises. A SOT (sensory organization test) is often ordered as well (Fig. 6).

Jaw-neck dysfunction was present in Sharon and she was referred for assessment and management by combined consultation of dentists as well as maxillo-facial unit staff. Our dentist performed a functional examination of the stomato-gnathic system, and the other unit arranged therapeutic jaw exercises for Sharon.

Changes were also detected in muscle activation patterns in this whiplash patient and arrangement was made for ambulant myofeedback training and forms the rationale of adding bio-feedback to our program (Voerman et al., Clin J Pain, 2006). We followed the strategy as suggested by Voerman, where feedback was provided whenever muscle relaxation was insufficient as the author does not use botox for this condition, although this has been reported recently in the literature. Trigger point injections sometimes do help ,however, and are done with the help of physiotherapist who helped the author to map out the points beforehand. In more difficult cases, muscle activation patterns were compared during rest, typing, and stress tasks by surface electromyography before commencement of therapy.

Rehabilitation of the deep longus capitus, longus colli, semispinalis cervicus, and segmental multifidus was stressed by recent researchers, but most cases already responded pretty well to the afore-mentioned programs (Conley et al., Spine, 1995; Mayoux-Benhamou et al., Surgical and Radiologic Anatomy, 1994).

Refractory Cases of Whiplash-related Injuries

Had Sharon's symptoms been refractory to the above, a trial of pulsed electromagnetic fields (PEMF) therapy, or medial branch block (followed possibly by elective radiofrequency lesioning if effective as reported recently by Prushansky et al. (J Neurosurg Spine, 2006) would have been prescribed. Although a recent meta-analysis (Conlin et al., Pain Res Manag, 2005) seems unsure of the efficacy of PEMF therapy, it is worth a trial in refractory cases as it is non-invasive.

Prognostic Factors

Recent multivariable analysis revealed eight prognostic factors associated with a negative outcome:

- Older age
- Female gender
- Increasing lag time between injury date and presentation for treatment
- Initial pain location

- Province of injury
- Higher initial pain intensity
- Lawyer involvement
- Being at work on entry to the clinic
- The effect of lawyer involvement was stronger for patients with less intense pain on initial visit (Dufton et al., Spine, 2006).

Learning Point

- In chronic whiplash-associated disorders patients can present with a myriad of symptoms, not just neck, shoulder and arm pain. These complex symptoms may involve jaw-neck motor control dysfunction, oculomotor and vestibular dysfunction, altered sensorimotor processing and muscle activation patterns, and even dysphagia.
- Since the above symptoms need dedicated specialists across different specialties, a multi-disciplinary team is frequently needed, especially for those patients who present late, despite the fact that some recent papers have challenged the use of multi-disciplinary teams.
- As for physical therapy, emphasis on the training of deep longus capitus, longus colli, semispinalis cervicus, and segmental multifidus is recommended (Conley et al., Spine, 1995; Mayoux-Benhamou et al., Surgical and Radiologic Anatomy, 1994), particularly those with only partial response despite treatment by the multi-disciplinary team.
- Techniques like PEMF and even radiofrequency neurotomy may be considered as a last resort. An occasional case may have the rehabilitation process hampered by on-going law suits and secondary gain issues that may affect prognosis.

References

1. Adams H, Ellis T, et al. (2007) Psychosocial factors related to return to work following rehabilitation of whiplash injuries. J Occup Rehabil, 17(2):305–15

2. Stewart MJ, Maher CG, et al. (2007) Randomized controlled trial of exercise for chronic whiplash-associated disorders. Pain, 128(1–2):59–68

3. Ferrantelli JR, Harrison DE, et al. (2005) Conservative treatment of a patient with previously unresponsive whiplash-associated disorders using clinical biomechanics of posture rehabilitation methods. J Manipulative Physiol Ther, 28(3):e1–8

4. Conlin A, Bhogal S, et al. (2005) Treatment of whiplash-associated disorders. I. Non-invasive interventions, Pain Res Manag, 10(1):21–32

5. Spitzer WO, Skovron ML, et al. (1995) Scientific monograph of the Quebec Task Force on Whiplash-Associated Disorders. Spine, 20:1S–73S

6. Stewart M, Maher CG, et al. (2007) Responsiveness of pain and disability measures for chronic whiplash. Spine, 32(5):580–5

7. Eriksson PO, Henrikson B, et al. (2007) Jaw-neck dysfunction in whiplash-associated disorders. Arch Oral Biol, 52(4):404–48

Sizable Cartilage Defect in a Professional Footballer

History and Examination

John is a 27-year-old professional footballer in the prime of his career, for he represents and has led his country to win many soccer matches. You got a call from your old friend Paul who is the athletics trainer of the football club to which John belongs because Paul is worried about the right knee of his top player. In the latest soccer match, John had persistent pain and on and off swelling of his right knee after a tackle from behind during the match. A radiograph was taken as arranged by the team physician and was passed as normal. The clinical notes of the team physician recorded no signs of cruciate, meniscal or collaterals injury. When you finally saw John the following week in your office, there was still mild effusion, and the range of motion was 5–125° for the right knee with a mild decrease in quadriceps bulk; otherwise you agreed with the clinical findings of the team physician. However, you did notice a subtle abnormality in the lateral radiograph of the right knee (Fig. 7). How would you proceed assuming that subsequent arthroscopy confirmed a 6-cm, full-thickness, cartilaginous defect at the trochlea of the right knee with no kissing lesion, no tibio-femoral mal-alignment, no evidence of arthrosis elsewhere and no sign of meniscal or cruciate ligament injury? John, in addition, asked about the likelihood of generalized arthrosis as a sequela of the lesion – what are your views?

Discussion

In general, most orthopods treat lesions less than or equal to 2 cm^2 using the micro-fracture technique. Cartilage defects up to 4 cm^2 can

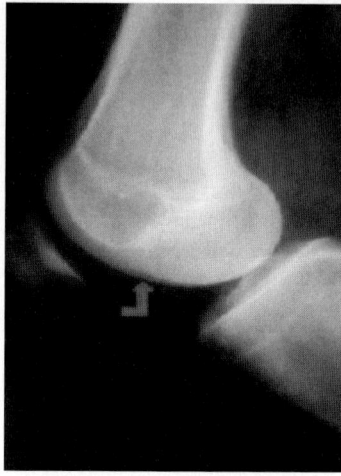

Fig. 7 The pointer in the lateral radiograph shows the cartilaginous lesion of the trochlea

sometimes be treated by the mosaic-type osteochondral autologous transplantation. Autologous chondrocyte implantation (ACI) should be considered when larger defects are presented in the younger patient. If there is already existing osteoarthritis, ACI is not recommended. Up till now, there has been no significant difference in outcomes comparing ACI and mosaicplasty or microfracture in the literature.

This case in question is a good indication of ACI since there is a focal, full-thickness, sizable chondral defect of the femoral trochlea, the age of the patient being between 15 and 50, the lesion is large (> 6 cm diameter), no generalized arthrosis, no bipolar disease or kissing lesion, and John is a motivated and compliant patient, with satisfactory gross lower limb alignment.

We can either proceed with the well-known ACI technique or the newer MACI (matrix-induced ACI), via the use of biological scaffolds such as type I/III collagen membrane to replace the traditional periosteum. The membrane is of porcine origin with a bi-layered structure, an outer flat layer with low friction and closely aggregated fibers, and an inner surface that is rough with a loose arrangement of collagen fibers presenting a larger surface area for chondrocyte adhesion. Electron microscopy done previously confirmed chondrocyte migration to this membranous scaffolding.

Following matching to the chondral defect, the chondrocyte seeded membrane will be secured by fibrin glue.

In a recent review of 63 patients with the defect covered with a type I/III collagen membrane, the ICRS and modified Cincinnati score showed significant improvement ($p < 0.01$) in all time intervals between preoperative and 6, 18, and 36 months after surgery. There was no significant difference in the final outcome between different defect localizations. Graft hypertrophy can be avoided by using a collagen membrane (Steinwachs et al., Arthroscopy, 2007).

Natural History

Mechanical injury is considered to be a major inductor of articular cartilage destruction and therefore a risk factor for the development of secondary osteoarthritis. Mechanical injury induces damage to the tissue matrix directly or mediated by chondrocytes via expression of matrix-degrading enzymes and reduction of biosynthetic activity.

It is too early, however, to say whether timely treatment of John's 6-cm lesion by ACI will alter the natural history. This is because the natural history of many chondral lesions has not been proven beyond doubt.

Rehabilitation Protocol Post-ACI for John

- Stage 1: Involves the immediate use of CPM allowing 0–40° initially, then gradually increase the range, brace is needed for protection in the early postoperative period to maintain joint mobility, as well as pain and edema control
- Stage 2: Involves protecting the joint against compression and shear forces of the injured area treated by ACI
- Stage 3: Involves a gradual loading phase – to provide the implanted chondrocytes the needed stimulus to hypertrophy and adapt in order to restore their natural function

Overall, the exercises and weight-bearing progression allowed is based on the size and features of the defect, but only touch-down weight-bearing is allowed in the initial 6 weeks, by the end of which we aim at an active ROM 0–90°.

Later in the course of rehabilitation, muscle strengthening commences and we also place stress on patient education. We expect the athlete to return to normal gait at around 3–6 months. But despite recent advances, most experts in the ACI technique noted at least 12–15 months if not more for cases with sizable lesions before these athletes are allowed to resume sporting events, and frequently only after second-look arthroscopy.

Monitoring the Newly Formed Tissue

- Follow-up arthroscopy is often used, but the one large drawback is that it shows the gross appearance only, which can sometimes be very deceiving.
- Newer techniques including the use of Atomic Force Microscopy, which can assess in detail the topography of bio-engineered cartilage. Thus, for the first time, atomic force microscopy was used to characterize surface topography of tissue-engineered cartilage (Romito et al., Ann Biomed Eng, 2006); meanwhile, special probes like Artscan can help assess the stiffness of the new surface.

Learning Point

- Understanding the biological functionality of the materials used in ACI requires reliable methods for structural imaging on the nano-scale – such as by atomic force microscopy, rather than its postoperative gross appearance on microscopy.
- The natural history of the full-thickness chondral defect has not been completely elucidated. However, the most popular techniques like microfractures, etc., are suitable only for chondral defects ≤2 cm^2 in size.

References

1. Steinwachs M, Kreuz PC, et al. (2007) Autologous chondrocyte implantation in chondral defects of the knee with a type I/III collagen membrane: A prospective study with a 3-year follow-up. Arthroscopy, 23(4):381–7

2. Romito L, et al. (2006) Mechanical interlocking of engineered cartilage to an underlying polymeric substrate: Towards a biohybrid tissue equivalent. Ann Biomed Eng, 34(5):737–47

Functional Knee Complaints in a Child with Cerebral Palsy

History and Examination

You met a child in the pediatric orthopedic outpatients department the other day, aged 8 years and called Mary. Mary was born premature and was noted to have a diplegic type of cerebral palsy and GMFCS level 2. Mary had previous bilateral ilio-psoas tenotomies and adductor releases, as well as distal medial hamstring lengthening nearly 2 years ago in another children's hospital. Mary's parents then moved to the state of Ohio where you work and, on examination, you noticed impaired right foot clearance in the swing phase of gait when Mary walked into your office; this was compensated for by voluntary contralateral vaulting, and some degree of external rotation of the leg. The mother told you that Mary nearly tripped over twice in the past month.

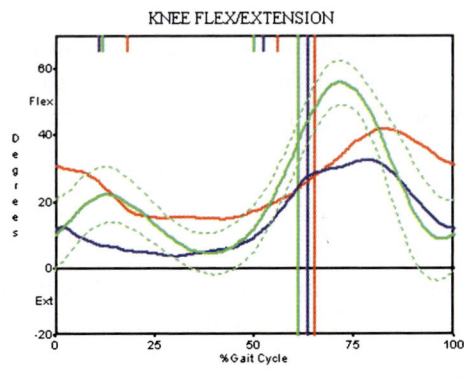

Fig. 8 Notice in the sagittal kinematics profile the delayed and reduced peak knee flexion in the swing phase of gait

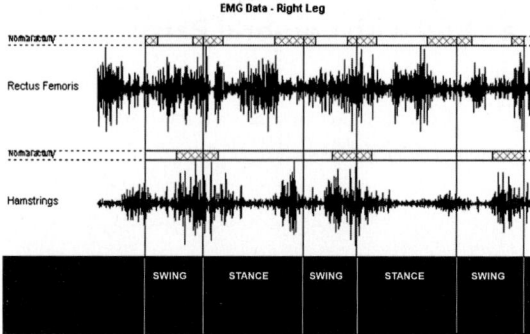

Fig. 9 Note the increased electromyography activity of the right rectus femoris muscle in swing

Further bedside examination revealed wearing of the toe platforms of her right shoe, the Duncan-Ely test proved to be positive. The ROM on the right side was affected and was only 70% of the normal range. Subsequent kinematics profile (Fig. 8) during gait analysis shows the typical pattern of a stiff knee gait: With swing-phase diminished peak knee flexion, and diminished slope of stance to swing flexion wave; while surface electromyography (EMG) studies revealed a prolonged and abnormal increase in the right rectus femoris activity during the swing phase (Fig. 9).

Elective right distal rectus transfer was performed with re-attachment of the tendon ends to semitendinosus.

Postoperatively, there was marked improvement in slope and magnitude of knee flexion in both late stance and early swing as reviewed by the kinematics profile. What benefits, if any, do you think preoperative gait analysis may help in the decision-making process regarding this child with a functional knee problem?

Discussion

Spasticity, muscle contracture formation, impairments of motor control, weakness, balance deficits, and extrapyramidal motions can all contribute to the functional limitations imposed at the knee. Careful clinical evaluation of the child and their gait must be performed in order to determine the best individual course of treatment. Often, three-dimensional motion analysis with assessment of muscle activity and force is necessary to completely assess the complexities of gait. Several typical gait patterns have been described involving the knee, including "jump knee," "crouch," "true equinus," "apparent equinus," "recurvatum," and "stiff knee" (Chambers, Eur J Neurol, 2001).

"Stiff knee gait" represents mainly a swing phase problem, featured by delayed and reduced knee flexion in swing, and frequently associated with compensations to aid leg clearance.

Commonly seen compensation strategies include circumduction, external rotation of the affected side, as well as contralateral vaulting. The etiology is frequently spasticity of the rectus femoris – often unmasked by previous distal hamstring lengthening.

The Ely test was shown to have a good positive predictive value (i.e., the certainty about the presence of rectus spasticity in patients with a positive Ely test result) for rectus femoris dysfunction during gait (Marks et al., Dev Med Child Neurol, 2003).

As for the role of gait analysis, it is most useful to have the preoperative EMG during gait analysis to confirm a spastic and overactive rectus femoris co-spasticity in swing before proceeding to surgery.

Most units perform rectus transfer medially to the medial hamstring – commonly semitendinosus – while at the same time lengthening the medial hamstring. Sewing the end of the rectus to the cut end of the semitendinosus gives greatest arm movement, and is preferred to simple distal release.

Proximal release is not effective unless the ROM of the affected side is > 80% normal, as shown by Sutherland. Thus, experts like Sutherland always perform a distal rectus transfer for most cases that go to surgery with a ROM of < 80% of the norm.

In addition, Chambers (a colleague of Sutherland's) showed previously that the procedure of rectus femoris transfer is effective *even* in the presence of co-contraction of both rectus and vastus lateralis in swing.

Learning Point

- "Stiff knee gait" represents mainly a swing phase problem, featured by delayed and reduced knee flexion in swing, and frequently associated with compensation to aid leg clearance.
- Dynamic EMG in gait analysis is most useful in confirming an abnormal rectus femoris muscle firing pattern in swing *before* we embark on surgery.
- Distal rectus transfer with re-attachment to the semitendinosus gives greatest arm movement, and is preferred against simple distal release or proximal release and represents the treatment of choice in most cases.

References

1.   Chambers HG (2001) Treatment of functional limitations at the knee in ambulatory children with cerebral palsy. Eur J Neurol., 8 Suppl 5:59–74
2.   Marks MC, Alexander J, et al. (2003) Clinical utility of the Duncan-Ely test for rectus femoris dysfunction during the swing phase of gait. Dev Med Child Neurol, 45(11):763–8

Hamstrings Injuries in a Professional Sprinter

History and Examination

Yesterday, you saw a 28-year-old professional athlete Elizabeth who specializes in sprinting and short putts, and has won several gold medals in the past. Six days ago, Elizabeth noticed sudden onset of pain and weakness during the explosive action of sprinting and heard an audible pop at the time of injury. There followed posterior right thigh pain near the beginning of the sporting event making her unable to continue to play. Besides pain, Elizabeth experiences a feeling of inadequate leg control and reports pain while sitting or walking up and down stairs, and she also noticed that her posterior thigh was bruised. Elizabeth attributed her right leg injury to lack of adequate warm-up. On examination, Elizabeth had pain with active knee flexion against resistance, performed with the hip in a neutral position and the knee in an extended starting position. You also palpated for tenderness at the ischial origin of her hamstrings in the prone position with the knee flexed at 90°. Next, in the supine position with hips flexed to 90°, you recorded the maximum tolerable active and passive knee extension angle and compared it with the contralateral leg. A subsequent radiograph did not reveal any bony avulsion, but a subsequent MRI showed an incomplete hamstring tear at the proximal myotendinous junction of the right leg. How would you proceed to manage Elizabeth's injuries?

Discussion

Hamstring injuries are the most prevalent muscle injury in sports that involve rapid acceleration, sprinting, and short putts. Injury typically occurs in an acute manner through an eccentric mechanism at the terminal stages of the swing phase of gait. The biceps femoris is the most commonly injured of the hamstrings. Re-injury rates are high and management is a challenge given the complex multi-factorial etiology. The high rates of hamstring injury and re-injury may result from a lack of high-quality research into the etiological factors underlying injury. Re-injury may also result from inaccuracy in diagnosis that results from the potential multi-factorial causes of these conditions (Thelen et al., Exerc Sport Sci Rev, 2006).

As pointed out by Hoskins, there has been a relative lack of high-quality research into the rehabilitation and prevention of hamstring injuries in the past as opposed to, say ACL injuries. As a result, an evidence-based approach to injury management is incomplete if not missing. Management in most units is based mainly on clinical experience, anecdotal evidence and the knowledge of the biological basis of tissue repair.

Hamstring injuries can be quite debilitating and often result in chronic problems. Eccentric muscle actions are often the last line of defense against muscle injury and ligament disruption, but traditionally, the focus of hamstring strength rehabilitation has been on concentric muscle actions. We will discuss this point further later on.

Clinical Diagnosis Vs. Use of MRI

A comparison between clinical assessment and magnetic resonance imaging of acute hamstring injuries has been reported recently in the literature.

Clinical and MRI assessments were in agreement in 38 out of 58 cases or 65% in a recent study in AJSM. In the same study, 31% had a clinically positive diagnosis, but no abnormalities were evident on MRI. In 3.4% of cases, MRI detected an injury, but the clinical examination had negative or equivocal findings.

Both clinical examination and MRI findings were strongly correlated with the actual time required to return to competition ($p < 0.001$ in both situations). This study reported in AJSM serves to show that MRI is *not* always required for estimating the duration of rehabilitation of an acute minor or moderate hamstring injury in professional football players (Svhneider-Kolsky et al., Am J Sports Med, 2006). That said, a recent Cochrane Review in 2007 pointed out that it is often impossible to differentiate between injuries of the muscle bellies and musculo-tendinous junctions based on a clinical assessment alone, thus the occasional indication for MRI.

Grades of Severity

- Grade One (first degree): Involves mild pain at the time (or within 24 h) of injury, especially when stress is applied to the injury. Local tenderness may or may not be present.
- Grade Two (second degree): Strains are present when the individual notices pain during activity and usually has to stop; pain and local tenderness are moderate to severe when the injury is stressed.
- Grade Three (third degree): Injury usually involves complete, or near complete, rupture or avulsion of at least a portion of a ligament or tendon with severe pain or loss of function; a palpable defect may be present (according to Kellett, 1986).

Etiology of Hamstring Injuries

Injuries to the hamstring muscles can be devastating because these injuries frequently heal slowly, have a tendency to recur, and preventive measures, as well as correction of the improper lumbo-pelvic hip posture, which is found in the majority of cases, is of paramount importance. It is thought that many of the recurrent injuries to the hamstring musculo-tendinous unit are the result of inadequate rehabilitation following the initial injury. The severity of hamstring injuries is usually of first or second degree, but occasionally third-degree injuries (complete rupture of the musculo-tendinous unit) do occur. Most hamstring strain injuries occur while running or sprinting, as in the present case scenario.

Thelen showed that peak hamstring stretch occurs during the late swing phase and is invariant with speed, but does depend on tendon compliance and the action of other muscles in the lumbo-pelvic region (Thelen et al., Exerc Sport Sci Rev, 2006).

Several etiological/predisposing factors have been proposed as being related to injury of the hamstring musculo-tendinous unit. They include: Poor flexibility, inadequate muscle strength and/or endurance, dyssynergic muscle contraction during running, insufficient warm-up and stretching prior to exercise, awkward running style, and a return to activity before complete rehabilitation following injury (Agre, Sports Med, 1985).

Main Treatment Modalities

Modalities often stressed by previous researchers include: PRICE (i.e., Protection, Rest, Ice, Compression and Elevation) exercise therapy to strengthen, stabilize and lengthen, including stretching (Croisier, 2002), and in fact some papers stressed the importance of the daily frequency of stretching although its importance was not confirmed in a recent *Cochrane Evidence Based Review* published in 2007. The said Cochrane review also mentioned that proper consideration should be given to the lumbar spine, sacro-iliac and pelvic alignment and postural control mechanisms while managing hamstring injuries. Other modalities include electrotherapy, with an alleged increase in healing rates (Van der Windt, 1999); massage therapy and mobilization was stressed by Brosseau and Hunter, and finally one should not forget the importance of functional rehabilitation before return to play.

Prevention Measures

Sherry in 2004 reported that those athletes performing a progressive agility and trunk stabilizing program presented with a significantly lower re-injury rate at both 2 weeks and 12 months following full return to sporting activity. Sherry recommended that participants continued their exercise programs at least three times a week for 2 months following this return. Sherry further suggested that the reduced incidence of recurrence could possibly be attributed to enhanced neuromuscular control of the lumbar spine and pelvis from where the hamstrings take attachment on the ischial tuberosity.

The importance of lumbar stability or core stability and pelvic motor control may also be factors in reducing the rate of recurrence of hamstring injury and was stressed in the recent Cochrane Systematic Review. The author usually emphasizes the importance of the training of the deep longitudinal system that includes the erector spinae muscle, the deep lamina of the thoraco-dorsal fascia, the sacro-tuberous ligament, and the biceps femoris muscle. Another area the author stresses includes postural training and re-establishment of the proper nutation of the pelvic girdle. It should be noted that the biceps femoris, for instance, can control the degree of sacral nutation via its connection to the sacro-tuberous ligament (Wingerden et al., 1993). Thus, in the author's view, improper pelvic girdle nutation can predispose to hamstring tears, while on the other hand people with a normal pelvic girdle to start with can end up with a "vertical" sacrum posture from highly overactive hamstrings that are extra tight.

In agreement with the author, researchers like Malliaropoulos found that concurrent changes in pelvic position and alignment are frequently identified in athletes with hamstring injuries, and proper correction of abnormal or altered pelvic alignment serves to relieve the stresses on structures that are involved in producing knee flexion, including the hamstrings. Cibulka even showed in as early as 1986, that *all* affected participants in his series presented with some form of mal-alignment of the lumbo-pelvic-hip complex, although he did not specifically emphasize the importance of having and/or restoring proper nutation of the pelvic girdle.

Period of Rehabilitation

Injuries to the tendinous or myotendinous junction are generally believed to take longer to rehabilitate than those in the muscle tissue (Garrett, 1984).

Higher grades of injury will take longer to rehabilitate due to the extent of damage to the tissues awaiting repair. It has been found in more severe cases that the convalescence interval prior to return to full activity can be longer than 6 weeks (Pomeranz, 1993).

The time taken for re-training can be significantly shorter in elite athletes as opposed to recreational athletes (Malliaropoulos, 2004).

Additional Rehabilitation Measures Used by the Author

Besides all the above-mentioned strategies, which will not be discussed again, the author includes the following in the rehabilitation protocol of hamstring injuries:

- Underwater walking, as frequently practiced in the Scandinavian countries
- Spine support device – sports-dependent, usually given to the athlete during under-water walking exercise in the initial stages
- Backward walking – included as part of the strategies used in functional rehabilitation
- Lumbo-pelvic stabilization – already mentioned
- Postural re-training – emphasis is on restoration of proper nutation of the pelvic girdle
- Frequency of stretching should in fact be individualized
- Progressive agility and trunk stabilization exercises, therapeutic ball exercises useful during functional rehabilitation
- Progressive resistance exercises and sports-specific training

New Development: Emphasis on Eccentric Training

- As already mentioned, traditionally, the focus of hamstring strength rehabilitation has been on concentric muscle actions.
- The result of the author echoed by many others like Kaminski, serves to illustrate the effectiveness of isotonic strength training on the development of hamstring muscle strength. More important is the dramatic effect of *eccentric strength training* on overall hamstring muscle strength, both isotonic and isokinetic. As pointed out by Kaminski, clinicians should consider using eccentric hamstring strengthening as part of their rehabilitation protocols for hamstring and knee injuries (Kaminski et al., J Athl Train, 1998).

Return to Play

- There are currently no consensus guidelines or agreed-upon criteria for safe return to sport following muscle strains that will completely eliminate the risk for recurrence and maximize performance; a similar view is shared by the Cochrane Review.

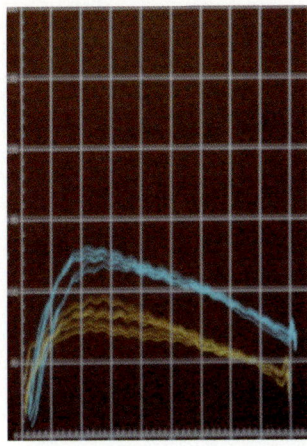

Fig. 10 In the isokinetic tracing, we find that the power of the right hamstrings (*yellow*) is weaker than the left (*blue*)

- Improved prognostic assessment of muscle strains with injury identification (MRI) and injury assessment (isokinetic testing – Fig. 10) may assist practitioners to lower, but not eliminate, recurrent injuries (Orchard et al., Clin J Sports Med, 2005).
- That said, another study showed that not even isokinetic strength testing can predict injury to hamstrings among footballers (Bennell, Wajswelner, et al., School of Physiotherapy, University of Melbourne).

Learning Point

- Treatment for hamstring injuries includes rest and immobilization immediately following injury and then a gradually increasing programme of mobilization, strengthening and activity, with emphasis on lumbo-pelvic-hip stabilization and restoration of proper sacral nutation.

■ Permission to return to play should be withheld until full rehabilitation has been achieved with complete return of muscle strength, endurance and flexibility in addition to a return
of co-ordination and athletic agility, and after a period of
functional followed by sports-specific rehabilitation. Failure
to achieve full rehabilitation will only predispose the athlete
to recurrent injury.

■ The best treatment for hamstring injuries is prevention, since
healing is slow; prevention should include training to maintain and/or improve strength, flexibility, endurance, co-ordination, agility, and the use of good postures, adequate warm-
up and warm-down.

■ Although most hamstring injuries can be treated conservatively, surgical management is recommended in cases when
two hamstrings with retraction >2 cm or three hamstrings
are avulsed from the ischial tuberosity (JAAOS 2007).

References

1. Mason D, et al. (2007) Rehabilitation for hamstring injuries. Cochrane Database Syst
    Rev, (1):CD004575
2. Orchard J, Best TM, et al. (2005) Return to play following muscle strains. Clin J
    Sports Med, 15(6):436–41
3. Agre JC (1985) Hamstring injuries. Proposed aetiological factors, prevention, and
    treatment. Sports Med, 2(1):21–33
4. Thelen DG, Chumanov ES, et al. (2006) Neuromusculoskeletal models provide in-
    sights into the mechanisms and rehabilitation of hamstring strains. Exerc Sport Sci
    Rev, 34(3):135–41
5. Hoskins W, Pollard H (2005) The management of hamstring injury. I. Issue in Diag-
    nosis. Man Ther, 10(2):96–107
6. Kaminski TW, Wabbersen CV, et al. (1998) Concentric versus enhanced eccentric
    hamstring strength training: Clinical implications. J Athl Train, 33(3):216–221
7. Cohen S, Bradley J (2007) Acute proximal hamstring rupture. JAAOS,
    15 (6):350–355

Was it Simply Tachycardia or Something More Sinister?

History and Examination

You were called by a staff nurse at midnight during a house call in an spinal cord injury (SCI) ward to attend to 39-year-old Jimmy who was found to have a pulse rate of 120/min, was sweating and generally unwell. Jimmy had suffered a complete cervical SCI in the past, was nursed at home with double incontinence, and recently admitted for a sacral sore to the SCI (spinal cord injury) ward.

Upon your arrival, Jimmy was found to have facial flushing, nasal stuffiness, hypertension, and anxiety. Subsequent urgent blood work was unremarkable, and urgent ECG showed a sinus tachycardia. There was neither fever nor rigors. Minutes later, the senior registrar arrived and asked immediately to check Jimmy's Foley catheter including any kinking and felt for any palpable bladder. The Foley was indeed kinked and Jimmy had some symptomatic relief after a new Foley was in place.

However, Jimmy was still feeling some generalized uneasiness with a mild tachycardia of 95/min when you did your morning rounds the next morning. You remembered your senior diagnosed autonomic dysreflexia yesterday, and did a per rectal examination with digital fecal evacuation. Jimmy's symptomatology eventually subsided completely thereafter.

Discussion

Autonomic dysreflexia is a known possible complication in SCI patients. It is characterized by acute hypertensive episodes, often triggered by some sensory stimulation below the level of injury. The chemicals involved in its pathogenesis include dopamine, dopamine-beta-hydroxy-lase and norepinephrine. These agents are released due to the stimulation of the (still intact) sympathetic neural tissue at the inter-medio-lateral gray matter below the level of SCI triggered by the ascending volleys of activation below. After SCI, the supraspinal centers cannot act to decrease the sympathetic response.

This syndrome is seen in cord lesions at/above T6 in the majority of cases (i.e., above the major T6–L2 sympathetic outflow). The hypertensive episodes cannot simply be controlled by the body's carotid or aortic receptors. A high index of suspicion is required in its diagnosis.

The symptomatology includes vasodilatation and sweating above the level of the SCI, and vasoconstriction and pallor below the level of SCI. The patient is mostly nervous and uneasy, with rising blood pressure and pounding headaches. Too high BP can even cause cerebral hemorrhage and death.

Suspect the diagnosis if there is a sudden increase in BP of 20–40 mmHg, or 15–20 mmHg in the adolescent. A systolic BP of 150 mmHg is regarded as a potentially dangerous level.

Precipitating Factors

In every case, it is essential to find out the underlying trigger of the episode. Common triggers include: Urinary related problems such as urinary retention, blocked Foley catheter, renal colic, or after cystoscopy procedures. Bowel-related problems such as fecal impaction. Other causes include GI causes like appendicitis, cholecystitis, thrombosed hemorrhoids, or even a rough per rectum examination or rough digital evacuation maneuver. Miscellaneous precipitating factors include pressure sores, heterotrophic ossification (HO), deep vein thrombosis (DVT)/phlebitis, in-growing toenails (IGTN), etc.

Management

Initial management involves putting the patient upright to reduce cerebral hyper-perfusion, loosen tight clothing, take off pressure stockings in the lower limb.

Other lines of management include Continuous BP monitoring every 5 min, identify and treat aforementioned triggers, as just described. If the Foley is blocked, either replace the Foley or if irrigation is attempted, do not use a large amount of fluid to irrigate, since bladder distension can cause a further rise in BP. Remember to use fluid at body temperature during irrigation, not cold fluids.

If unresponsive to the above measures, consider anti-hypertensive agents, e.g., nitroglycerine, nifedipine and/or prazosin, hydralazine. Nifedipine can be administered by the bite and swallow method for its prompt action, avoid the (erratic absorption) sublingual route.

For cases in which dysreflexia was triggered by existing bowel program, one may consider prophylactic medication such as captopril.

Learning Point

- A high index of suspicion is needed to diagnose autonomic dysreflexia.
- Front line medical and nursing staff should be taught about the first aid measures to reduce cerebral hyper-perfusion to prevent complications like cerebral hemorrhage or even death.
- Underlying trigger(s) in individual cases always need to be identified and promptly corrected to prevent recurrence.

References

1. Consortium for Spinal Cord Medicine, Clinical Practice Guidelines (website of paralyzed veterans of America)
2. Ip D (2007) Orthopedic rehabilitation, assessment, and enablement. Springer, chapter 12

History and Examination

You got a referral from the family physician of a 42-year-old secretary Helen, who suffers from intractable right-sided inferior heel pain, particularly with the first few steps that she takes in the morning. She had difficulty waiting for the bus to go to her work-place. She had got to the point now of walking on her toes to avoid the terrible heel pain.

Initially, the pain tended to decrease with level ground ambulation, but now it has increased throughout the day. The pain is worsened by walking barefoot on hard surfaces or by walking upstairs. She did not notice any numbness or weakness.

Helen believed that her symptoms started after chasing after buses on several occasions when she was late getting up in the morning for work, coupled with a recent change in the type of shoe wear.

On physical examination, you found that Helen was obese, and tender to palpation at the antero-medial aspect of the right heel. You also noticed some ankle dorsiflexion tightness arising from the Achilles tendon.

Her pain was exacerbated by passive dorsiflexion of the toes. There was no clinical evidence of enthesopathy, the heels were neutral, and there were no pes cavus or pes planus. There was no clinical suspicion of tarsal tunnel syndrome.

According to her referring doctor, Helen had received conventional treatment including all the modalities listed below for her right heel, but failed to show improvement. The therapy she had previously received included advice to decrease weight-bearing activities and running, shoe inserts and heel pads, and night splints made to hold the ankle in dorsiflexion and the toe in extension. Plantar fascia stretching was also previously being prescribed by a local physiotherapist, who also administered ultrasound treatment to the affected area.

How would you proceed from here?

Discussion

Pain that is worse on first arising in the morning or after a period of rest is highly suggestive of plantar fasciitis, as is typical local tenderness at the point of attachment of the plantar fascia at the medial tubercle of the calcaneus. Risk factors include weight gain, repetitive stress, and middle age. Our patient at hand in fact has most of the risk factors. The plantar fascia extends longitudinally along the plantar surface of the foot, deep to the fibrofatty subcutaneous tissue and covers the intrinsic musculature and neurovascular structures. Tensile forces are concentrated at this attachment site, particularly on the medial tubercle of the calcaneus.

Pathologic studies carried out more recently on surgically removed specimens demonstrate microtears of the fascia, collagen necrosis, angiofibroblastic hyperplasia, and chondroid metaplasia (JAAOS, 2006).

These changes are consistent with a chronic degenerative/reparative process secondary to repetitive stress or sometimes repeated microtrauma. The latter is evidenced by the frequent occurrence of heel pain in runners. The condition is bilateral in one-third of cases; a spur is present in half of all cases, as opposed to 15% in the general population. For bilateral cases, seronegative arthritis also needs to be ruled out.

One possible source of pain may be a branch of the lateral plantar nerve. Anatomically, the first branch of the lateral plantar nerve is a mixed motor-sensory nerve to the abductor digiti quinti minimi, which passes superior to the attachment of the plantar fascia. Authors like Baxter have drawn attention to a possible impingement syndrome that can occur in several areas along the course of this nerve (OCNA, 1989).

The spur, however, need not necessarily be the source of the pain, for it is well accepted that even though a spur may be seen coincidentally or even associated with the clinical condition, it need not by itself be the etiologic factor.

That said, there is a chance the spur might add to neurogenic pain with compression of the first branch of the lateral plantar nerve mentioned above (OCNA, 1989).

Most surgeons and physiatrists treat plantar fasciitis conservatively. Taping is mentioned in the podiatry literature, but has not been evaluated scientifically with regard to plantar fasciitis. Shoe modification, such as use of a steel shank to limit MTPJ dorsiflexion during toe-off or a heel lift, and a change to wearing high-heeled shoes to decrease heel impact have also been tried with variable success.

It is surprising that in a recent review article on the subject by Gill, the use of newer modalities like shockwave and magnetopulse therapy were not even mentioned. The author in fact found the use of shockwave therapy to be very useful in patients refractory to conventional physical therapy and shoewear modification.

Role of Shockwave Therapy

The use of shockwave therapy for the management of heel pain was formally approved by the FDA in 2000 (Fig. 11). The mechanism of action is not known for certain, but possibly involves controlled internal fascial disruption that may initiate a healing response.

Low-energy shockwave treatment is preferred to high-energy treatments. High-energy shockwave treatments may produce side-effects in the form of periosteal detachments and even small fractures on the inner surface of the cortex.

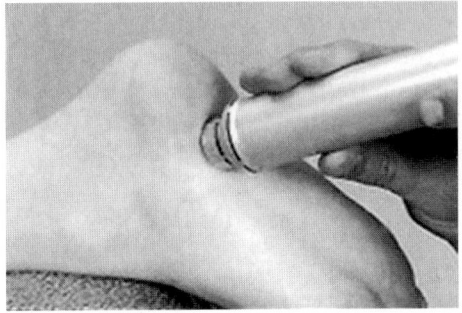

Fig. 11 Application of low-energy shockwave for plantar fasciitis

Pitfalls in Administering Shockwave Therapy

- First, make sure the side effects have subsided before the next treatment. In patients with a low pain threshold, operating pressure can be started at 2 bar and an operating frequency of 3 Hz. An analgesic effect sets in at approximately 500 pulses. As treatment continues, the pressure output and frequency can be increased to the recommended parameters.

- Finally, with the increased popularity of endoscopic plantar fascia release, there is concern regarding the overzealous and inappropriate use of a technique with known risks of nerve damage. To tackle the above risks, refer to the AAOS position statement on the role of surgery in heel pain: Suggesting the use of bone scan to confirm the diagnosis *before* proceeding to surgery, particularly since 90% of cases do respond to conservative treatment.

Learning Point

- The pathogenesis of plantar fasciitis is still not completely understood.
- However, there is increasing literature to support the use of newer modalities like shockwave therapy in the management of recalcitrant cases.
- Despite the enthusiasm of the endoscopic surgical option, the risks to the neural structures involved was heeded in the recent AAOS position statement.
- For patients who are irresponsive to conventional and shockwave therapy, the author will also try steroid iontophoresis (see Fig. 12) via the use of electricity or ultrasound before subjecting patients to surgical treatment, the administration of which follows guidelines as set out in the study by Gudeman et al. (ASJM, 1997).

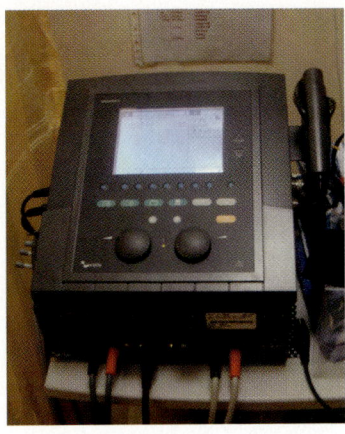

Fig. 12 Machine for the application of iontophoresis treatment

References

1. Rompe J-D (2002) Shock wave applications in musculoskeletal disorders. Thieme, Stuttgart
2. Sems A, Dimeff R, et al. (2006) Extracorporeal shockwave therapy in the treatment of chronic tendinopathy. J Am Acad Orthop Surg, 14:195–204
3. Maier M, Steinborn M, et al. (2000) Extracorporeal shockwave application for chronic plantar fasciitis associated with heel spurs: Prediction of outcome by magnetic resonance imaging. J Rheumatol, 27(10):2455–62
4. Gudeman SD, Eisele SA, et al. (1997) Treatment of plantar fasciitis by iontophoresis of 0.4% dexamethasone: A randomized double-blind, placebo controlled study. ASJM, 25(3):312–6
5. Carter R, Anderson, et al. (2003) Effects of iontophoresis current magnitude and duration on dexamethasone deposition and localized drug retention. Phys Ther, 83(2): 161–169

Hip Swelling after Combined TBI and SCI

History and Examination

You were asked to see a patient, Joseph, a 38-year-old engineer who suffered from both near complete cervical cord injury at C7 as well as traumatic brain injury (TBI) 4 months ago as a result of road traffic accident. The staff nurse noted left hip swelling during a change of bed sheets in the SCI ward. On examination, you found there was left hip fullness with decreased motion in all directions, and ordered a radiograph. There were no sign of sepsis or hernia, and the X-ray did not reveal any fracture, but signs of heterotopic ossification (HO) around the left hip. Serial X-rays confirmed HO, as did a subsequent CT scan (Fig. 13). Describe your subsequent management and what causes the diffuse hip swelling.

Discussion

Management starts with the use of gentle passive ROM exercises to chart and maintain available hip joint motion and to avoid contractures. In this case, since HO has already set in, a trial of intravenous bisphosphonates can be considered. Etidronate, being an analogue of first generation of bisphosphonates, has inhibitory actions on mineralisation and hydroxyapatite crystal formation, and is therefore commonly now used as a drug to treat ectopic ossification in cases of total hip arthroplasty and spinal cord injury. The effect of bisphosphonates in preventing calcification could be associated with the physical property to attach tightly to hydroxyapatite crystals in bone matrix (Ono and Wada, Clin Calcium, 2004).

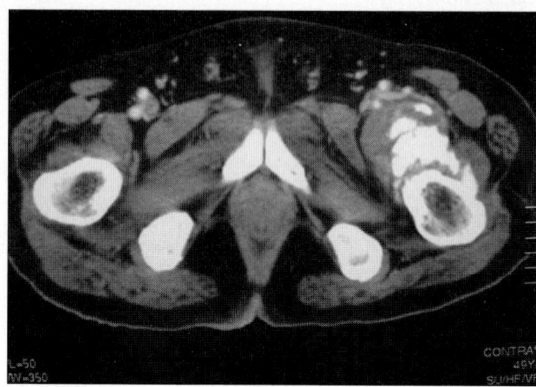

Fig. 13 Transverse CT cut showing the heterotopic ossification process developing around the left hip

C-reactive protein (CRP) needs monitoring while on etidronate treatment. The normalization of CRP is usually seen during the first 3–4 weeks of etidronate therapy, indicating a resolution of acute phase inflammatory reaction.

Serial radiological assessment and serial checking of alkaline phosphatase with or without CT are recommended. Nowadays, the Alonzo CT classification is preferred to the radiological Brook's classification since it makes the assessment in 3-D and not 2-D as conclusions drawn from 2-D simple radiographs can be misleading.

If ankylosis seems inevitable despite exercises, it is best for the patient if it occurs in the most functional position.

In general, surgery for removal of ectopic bone should be undertaken only for clear functional goals, such as improved standing posture or ambulation or independent dressing and feeding. Surgery is not usually undertaken earlier than 18 months after injury. In the current instance, our patient Joseph has tetraplegia and as long as the hip remains in the functional position, surgery is best avoided. As for the left hip fullness in this patient, it is likely to be partly due to heterotopic bone and partly due to local effusion, which was indeed confirmed by subsequent MRI. Effusion if present is most likely the result of repetitive microtrauma. Patients with paralysis are in general susceptible to effusions of the hip similar to those seen in documented cases regarding the knee joint, which are even more common (J Spin Cord Med, 2006).

Nature of HO

Heterotopic ossification (HO) is a condition characterized by the formation of extra-osseous bone in soft tissue frequently surrounding peripheral joints in patients after musculoskeletal trauma (e.g., after elbow fracture), or extensive surgical dissection (e.g., after total joint surgery or acetabular fracture surgery) or in some neurological conditions such as spinal cord injury (SCI) or traumatic brain injury (TBI), as in the present case scenario. Isolated HO can occur at any age, but is rare in the very young. Post-traumatic HO is common in young athletic persons. HO has been found to affect young patients with SCI more frequently, as in our patient.

The term heterotopic ossification has largely replaced myositis ossificans in the literature, but the term myositis ossificans traumatica can be applied to HO occurring after trauma or burns.

Early Diagnosis

Many clinicians rely on early detection of HO using triple-phase technetium Tc99 bone scanning, which detects early increases in vascularity and is a reliable indicator in making a diagnosis. The first and second phases of the triple-phase bone scan usually show increased uptake. The optimal timing is often quoted as roughly 3–4 weeks following the injury.

There are now recent reports of the use of MRI that can potentially identify the HO process even earlier still. Via the use of fast spin-echo short time inversion-recovery (STIR) images a so-called "lacy pattern" of the muscles in the peri-articular area can be discerned. The most affected part of the muscle group usually exhibits homogeneous high signal. Contrast-enhanced fat-suppressed T1-weighted images may also show a "lacy-like pattern" (Crit Care, 2006).

The use of ultrasound is mentioned occasionally in the literature, but ultrasound is not generally used to assess HO any more *after* the diagnosis is established, although some authors have proposed the use of ultrasound as a simultaneous screening tool for HO and DVT in patients with spinal cord injury.

Within hours of the onset of clinical symptoms, ultrasound may demonstrate chaotic disruption of the normal lamellar structure of skeletal muscle, which can be seen up to 10–14 days before radiographic evidence of HO. Later on, a zonal mass-like pattern develops that is peripherally echogenic and centrally hypoechoic. Radiographic visibility improves once mineralization sets in. In florid cases, ultrasound can demonstrate sheets of echogenic material with acoustic shadow. Findings of HO on ultrasound images should be confirmed with radiographs and followed up just as for other HO cases.

Histology
Serial histologic changes of HO following trauma begins with spindle cell proliferation within the first week, then primitive osteoid develops at the periphery of the lesion by 7–10 days. Primitive cartilage and woven bone tend to occur in the second week, with trabecular bone forming at 2–5 weeks. At the 6-week mark, a zonal phenomenon can be seen with central, immature tissues and mature lamellar bone peripherally.

Pathogenesis
An interesting new finding in basic science is that muscle tissue was recently demonstrated to show osteogenetic competence in response to osteo-inductive stimuli. The recent discovery of muscle-derived stem cells (MDSC) that can differentiate into an osteogenic lineage suggests not only that skeletal muscle can act as a source of osteoprogenitor cells, but might also be a plausible mechanism somewhere in the pathogenetic pathway for the production of HO.

Using a relatively new technology known as "RNA interference" to turn off genes that regulate cell differentiation, University of Pittsburgh researchers have demonstrated that they can increase the propensity of muscle-derived stem cells (MDSCs) to become bone-forming cells. Based on these results, the investigators believe that by turning off specific genetic factors they can control the capacity of MDSCs as a means of treating various musculoskeletal diseases and injuries.

Heterotopic ossification occurs in 25% of spinal cord injury patients, and in 20% of these the pathologic process is severe enough to cause limitations in joint motion.

Vascular and metabolic changes resulting from autonomic nervous system impairment may play a role in the etiology of HO (Da Paz et al., Med Hypotheses, 2007). A recent postulate has it that HO in patients with injury to the CNS may be related to a dysfunction of proprioception. With interruption of the neural tract of a given limb, ligaments lose control and coordination of their proprioceptive function and begin to react to direct stimuli in an independent, isolated and haphazard way. Free of CNS control and directly stimulated by such independent signals, mesenchymal osteoprogenitor cells located in soft tissues begin to occasion tissue maturation and differentiation into bone: Heterotopic bone (Da Paz et al., Med Hypotheses, 2007).

Management

The mainstay of management has already been mentioned. In the setting of total hip arthroplasty, Kocia et al. showed in 2006 that early treatment with PEMF (pulsed electro-magnetic fields) could prevent severe HO and reduce the overall HO. The mechanism of which is possibly to improve local tissue oxygenation, this is because some theories presume that local hypoxia of the soft tissue might cause HO. Whether the same can be applicable to other settings like SCI or TBI is unknown.

As for prophylaxis, besides the use of radiotherapy (with its side effects), there are recent reports that celecoxib seems more effective than ibuprofen in HO prophylaxis in the setting of total hip replacement (Saudan et al., J Bone Joint Surg Br, 2007).

Traditional teachings have advocated that PROM (passive range of motion exercises) is a contraindication when HO is present because it can lead to the development or exacerbate the formation of HO. A review of the literature only reveals a few scientific studies that concluded that forcible manipulation of stiff joints can lead to myositis ossification.

Most of the articles that have concluded that PROM is contraindicated were based on anecdotal findings. This conclusion is misleading as it is unfair for one to equate forcible manipulation of a joint as being synonymous with PROM exercises. Gentle PROM exercises in fact should be maintained in the body part affected by HO in most cases.

Lastly, there is some recent literature by Kocia concerning the role of PEMF treatment. Early use of pulsed electromagnetic fields (PEMF) could prevent this ossification since it accelerates the circulation and oxygenation of soft tissue. According to the results obtained, early treatment with PEMF could prevent severe HO and reduce overall HO.

Learning Point

- On pathophysiology: The discovery of the osteogenic potentials of muscle-derived stem cells hold promise of a better understanding of HO and should provide a rich field of further research, amid a host of other hypotheses.
- On earlier diagnosis: The use of MRI has the prospect of diagnosing HO even earlier than the bone scan awaiting further confirmation in future studies. Notice that radiographs cannot detect the mineralization of HO during the first 1–2 weeks after onset of symptoms or inciting trauma. Neither radiographs nor CT should be performed in the pelvic region during pregnancy.
- On management: A common pitfall is the misconception that "even passive ROM exercises should be avoided", which is untrue, as discussed.
- On prophylaxis: Celecoxib emerges as being a more promising pharmacological agent than non-selective NSAIDs in recent prospective randomized trials.

References

1. Ip D (2007) Orthopedic rehabilitation, assessment, and enablement. Springer, Chap 12

2. Kirshblum SC, Priebe MM, et al. (2007) Spinal cord injury medicine. III. Rehabilitation phase after acute spinal cord injury. Arch Phys Med Rehabil, 88 3 Suppl 1: S62–70

3. Argyropoulou MI, Kostandi E, et al. (2006) Heterotopic ossification of the knee joint in intensive care unit patients: Early diagnosis with magnetic resonance imaging. Crit Care, 10(5):R152

4. Ono K, Wada S (2004) Regulation of calcification by bisphosphonates. Clin Calcium, 14(6):60–3

5. Saudan M, Saudan P, et al. (2007) Celecoxib versus ibuprofen in the prevention of heterotopic ossification following total hip replacement: A prospective randomized trial. J Bone Joint Surg Br, 89(2):155–9

6. Da Paz AC, Carod Artal FJ (2007) The function of proprioceptors in bone organization: A possible explanation for neurogenic heterotopic ossification in patients with neurological damage. Med Hypotheses, 68(1):67–73

7. Kupfer M, Dholakia M (2006) Effusion of the hips in a patient with tetraplegia, J Spinal Cord Med, 29(2):160–2

Consultation for a Third Opinion on Bone Health

History and Examination

Elizabeth is a 45-year-old senior company secretary. She has all along had diffuse musculoskeletal aches and pains. As she feared osteoporosis after reading a newspaper article, she went to see her family physician, who ordered a DXA scan of the lumbar spine and hip. She was told that she had a T-score reading of −2.0 at the hip and that she does not yet have osteoporosis, at most osteopenia.

She subsequently went to see a private orthopedic surgeon who labeled her as having "borderline osteoporosis" and that he was prepared to offer her special drug treatment, essentially one of the bisphosphonates. Feeling very confused, she came to you for a third expert opinion with the DXA report in her hand. What will be your subsequent management of the patient?

Discussion

The WHO international reference standard for osteoporosis diagnosis is a T-score of −2.5 or less at the femoral neck. The reference standard from which the T-score is calculated is the female, white, age 20–29 years (NHANES III database).

The WHO classification should *not* be applied to healthy premenopausal women or healthy men under age 50; and in fact the use of Z-scores, *not* T-scores is preferred. This is particularly important in children. A Z-score of −2.0 or lower is defined as "below the expected range for age" and a Z-score above −2.0 is "within the expected range for age".

Osteoporosis may be diagnosed if there is low BMD based on Z-scores coupled with secondary causes (e.g., glucocorticoid therapy, hypogonadism, hyperparathyroidism, etc.).

In other words, the diagnosis of osteoporosis in healthy premenopausal women or healthy men under the age of 50 should *not* be made on the basis of densitometric criteria alone.

The Z-score Reference Database should, in addition, be population-specific where adequate reference data exist.For the purpose of Z-score calculation, the patient's self-reported ethnicity should therefore be used.

In summary, before one can properly manage this case, one should be aware that the WHO criteria for the diagnosis of osteoporosis apply only to post-menopausal Caucasian women, and is not directly applicable to a pre-menopausal lady.

In fact, the modern tendency nowadays, as far as osteoporosis is concerned, is to calculate and assess risk factors rather than treating a number (bone mass) per se. As far as risk factors go, maternal history of fragility fracture, past history of such fractures and the *age* of the patient is very important. In fact, to quote from the most recently published WHO guideline article on the use of BMD vs. risk factors: "…BMD shows limited validity in predicting fracture risk. A research group of the World Health Organization (WHO) has developed absolute risk assessment models for fracture incorporating several clinical risk factors with and without BMD" (Iki, Clin Calcium, 2007).

Also, dwelling on the issue of level of risk, *age* is a very significant factor. Thus, the significance we attach to the *same* T-score reading for a 60-year-old lady is very different from that of an 80-year-old lady.

Screening can be done if indicated for secondary causes especially if the Z-score turns out to be low. A biochemistry work-up is never complete without checking the blood levels of Ca P, thyroid function, 1,25-diOH vitamin D level, ALP and, where indicated, 24-h urinary calcium excretion. A hematological screen should also be included in older women. It is good news that the WHO just issued some guidelines or, in fact, more appropriately, viewpoints, concerning secondary osteoporosis, quoted as follows: "…In patients with osteoporosis caused by primary hyperparathyroidism, hyperthyroidism, diabetes mellitus as well as hormone deprivation therapy, bisphosphonate is effective in increasing bone mineral density but no data have been available about the fracture risk. Guidelines on the management and treatment of each secondary osteoporosis are desirable…" (Yamauchi, Clin Calcium, 2007).

In the present case, Elizabeth turns out indeed to have a low Z-score; she was found to have a low calcium diet, and the serum level of 1,25 di-OH Vitamin D was only 30% of the normal level. Calcium supplements and a loading dose of vitamin D was given, and she will be scheduled for a repeat Z-score six months later, as well as monitoring of serial bone turnover markers. Elizabeth was also found to have a high resting pulse rate, her free T4 was normal, but free T3 was elevated and she was referred to an endocrinology unit for management of her occult thyrotoxicosis.

Learning Point

- The popular WHO criteria for "diagnosis" of osteoporosis does not in fact apply to pre-menopausal women. In fact, the WHO has just issued multiple renewed guidelines basing on the calculation of risk factor instead, i.e., instead of placing stress on a number.
- Where densitometry studies are planned, the Z-scores need to be used instead in pre-menopausal ladies.
- Occult thyrotoxicosis is an important, readily treatable cause of secondary osteoporosis. This point was highly stressed in other publications by the author. So, it is interesting to note that in a recent review article on "secondary osteoporosis" published in *JAAOS*, 2007, this important, readily treatable cause was in fact not being stressed enough. WHO now favours the issue of guidelines for many different secondary causes of osteoporosis in the future.

■ If, for some reason, an orthopod wishes to consider bisphos-phonates in pre-menopausal ladies like the lady here, he should be aware that bisphosphonates have been shown to cause fetal harm in animals, but there are no data on the risk to the fetus in humans. Bisphosphonates should be used during pregnancy only if the orthopod feels that its potential benefit justifies the potential risk to the fetus. It is therefore usually contraindicated to give bisphosphonates to pre-menopausal ladies who desire to become pregnant.

References

1.   Position statement of the International Society of Clinical Densitometry 2005 Vancouver Conference
2.   Marqusee E, Haden ST (1998) Subclinical thyrotoxicosis, Endocrinol Metab Clin North Am, 27(1):37–49
3.   Iki M (2007) Absolute risk for fracture and WHO guideline: WHO model for assessing absolute risk of fracture. Clin Calcium, 17(7):1015–21
4.   Yamauchi M (2007) Absolute risk for fracture and WHO guideline: Treatment in patients with secondary osteoporosis.Clin Calcium, 17(7):1106–13

Was It Really Another Case of "Tennis Elbow"?

History and Examination

Jane is a 38-year-old right-handed computer worker who was referred to your office with a diagnosis of right tennis elbow diagnosed by a general practitioner and treated with a brief course of ultrasound, but to no avail. Physical examination at the elbow demonstrated neither direct tenderness over the anterior aspect of the lateral epicondyle nor its posterior and inferior aspect. Resisted wrist dorsiflexion, especially with the elbow extended, is often regarded as the most sensitive indirect maneuver, but was unremarkable. The radial-capitellar joint was assessed by direct palpation with pronation/supination and flexion/extension and was also normal. The lateral antebrachial cutaneous nerve evaluated as it passed the lateral margin of the biceps tendon was also normal. Postero-lateral rotatory instability of the elbow was also ruled out. Finally, the most plausible primary local differential diagnosis (radial tunnel syndrome) was assessed by anterior local tenderness along the radial nerve in the interval between the brachioradialis and brachialis as well as at the level of the radial neck.In this case, direct tenderness was present over the radius at 5 cm distal to the lateral epicondyle in full supination and was markedly greater than in pronation. The so-called middle finger test was also positive. Describe your subsequent management.

Discussion

The physical examination in this patient does not correspond to the typical tenderness expected in a case of lateral epicondylitis, and a positive middle finger test points more to the diagnosis of radial tunnel syndrome.

Radiographic evaluation will reveal epicondylar calcification in 5–20% of cases of real tennis elbow, but this is not prognostically related and is not indicated in this case.

MRI is useful in inconsistent cases, especially in secondary gain concerns, but its accuracy varies. The role of MRI in suspected radial tunnel syndrome has not been proven beyond doubt.

However, diagnostic lidocaine injection may be useful in more complex cases of possible concomitant pathologies or suspected isolated radial tunnel syndrome for confirmation of diagnosis.

A lidocaine block (6 cc of 2% lidocaine) at the radial tunnel, just proximal to the radial capitellar joint, may be used to substantiate radial neuropathy (J. Nunley, MD, Durham, NC, personal communication, 1990).

This patient in fact had had a course of conventional physiotherapy prior to being seen by a private practitioner and labeled as having some kind of tennis elbow. As expected, there was little to no effect on our patient's symptoms.

In this case, Jane had relief of her symptoms with the above-mentioned lidocaine injection and a diagnosis of radial tunnel was obtained. Her symptoms were relieved by subsequent decompression.

Recent studies in a rat model have indicated that the pathophysiologic mechanisms underlying development of work-related musculoskeletal disorders include widespread inflammation and subsequent fibrosis at high levels of repetition and force. A systemic inflammatory component may affect tissues not directly involved in task performance, thereby contributing to widespread and puzzling symptoms that are often characteristic of patients with such disorders (Barr et al., Exerc Sport Sci Rev, 2004). But whether the pathogenesis is founded on a similar basis in radial tunnel syndrome as opposed to lateral epicondylitis remains uncertain.

In general, physical risk factors of repetitive stress injury were found to be related to repetition, duration, working in awkward and static positions and forceful movements of the upper extremity and neck (Reneman, J Occup Rehabil, 2005), but again, whether these same factors that often contribute to the development of lateral epicondylitis also contribute to development in cases of radial tunnel syndrome is uncertain.

Learning Point

- One should not jump to the immediate conclusion of labeling a patient as having "tennis elbow" without carefully examining for the various differential diagnoses, for the other diagnoses have differences in treatment and prognoses.
- A lidocaine test may be helpful if unsure of the diagnosis in the case of suspected radial tunnel syndrome.

References

1. AAOS Instructional Course Lectures, vol 47, 1998, p 165
2. Barr AE, Barbe MF, et al. (2004) Systematic inflammatory mediators contribute to widespread effects in work-related musculoskeletal disorders. Exerc Sport Sci Rev, 32(4):135–42

A Patient Requesting an "Oxford Uni" for his knee OA

History and Examination

Mr Shum is a 60-year-old retired Chinese gentleman who used to be a trader in a local English trading company. He came to your office one day with a referral letter from his family physician, who wrote that Mr Shum is mainly having pain in the medial compartment of his right knee and that prior radiographs did not demonstrate significant degenerative changes in the patella-femoral articulation nor the lateral tibio-femoral compartment. Mr Shum has heard quite a few of his English friends talking about the excellent results they had after the Oxford uni-compartmental knee replacement, and wishes to seek your opinion on this score since the medial joint line pain has been getting worse by the day and he promised himself to do something about it. According to Mr Shum, the physiotherapy sessions he received in the past failed to relieve him of his suffering for the past 4 whole months. On examination, there was reasonable quadriceps bulk and minimal right genu varum and the left knee has good alignment. The Lachman test was negative and the collaterals stress test and McMurray tests were negative. The left knee has full motion range, and the right knee's range was 0–115°. You did a preoperative arthroscopy that helped confirm mainly medial compartment osteoarthritis of the right knee with significant degenerative changes, mainly in the central and posterior aspect of the right tibial condyle. Would you have proceeded with a uni-compartmental knee arthroplasty? And if so, will you pursue the model as requested by the patient, i.e., Oxford uni-compartmental replacement?

Discussion

Given the age and that your previous knee arthroscopy confirmed mainly uni-compartmental osteoarthritis, and that the retired Mr Sham does not make high demands on his knee, the decision of this patient to go for a uni-compartmental knee replacement seems to be a fair choice. The advantages of uni-compartmental knee replacement over total knee replacement (TKR) includes the preservation of soft tissue as well as bone stock, and better function with improved range of motion and more natural gait, and the Oxford Knee has been shown to preserve near normal patello-femoral mechanics (JBJS Br, 2006). However, patients should be made aware of the lower survival of the uni-compartmental knee replacement compared with total knee arthroplasties (Acta Orthop, 2007).

However, one should not forget about *ethnic* differences in the pattern of osteoarthritis, which has all along seldom been highlighted in the literature on implant selection when one contemplates using uni-compartmental knee replacement. According to David Murray of Oxford for instance, the successful Oxford Uni-compartmental knee replacement and its design are based on the observation that many Caucasians' knees have mainly antero-medial OA.

According to the latest study conducted at multiple centers in the People's Republic of China as well as Australia involving a total of 238 patients of Chinese and Caucasian ethnic origin whose patterns of knee OA were analyzed, Chinese patients have significantly greater wear at the central and posterior regions of the medial tibial condyle, just like what was seen in the radiograph of this patient preoperatively. This is in contrast with the Caucasians recruited to the study from Australia where antero-medial wear represents the common OA knee pattern (ORS Proceedings, 2007).

After discussion with the patient, another type of uni-compartmental knee implant was performed (Fig. 14) and Mr Shum made a speedy recovery on programmed rehabilitation involving early pre-emptive analgesia, adequate perioperative pain control, early full weight-bearing exercises, and early discharge on Day 5 with arrangements made for Mr Shum to return to day hospital for continuous ambulatory training and rehabilitation.

It is the author's belief that an implant is good in as much as it is implanted in the right patient with the right pathology. Although the Oxford uni-compartmental knee replacement has strong literature support, careful patient selection is needed, including analyzing the pathology at hand, which is important as illustrated by the current case scenario. Manufacturers of orthopedic implants, be it for joint replacement, fracture surgery, etc., should always take into account ethnic differences in both anatomy and pathology. On this score, the fact that experts like Bernard Morrey and co-workers are in the process of preparing re-sized extra-small implants for the smaller built Asian population in connection with their well-known Coorad-Morrey total elbow replacement is setting a good example for others to follow.

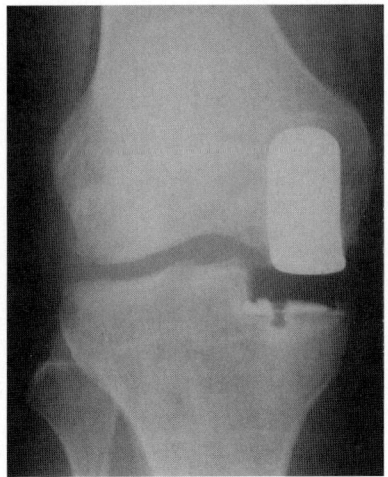

Fig. 14 Postoperative right knee radiograph after uni-compartmental knee replacement

Learning Point

■ The recent realisation of the effect of different ethnicity on the pattern of OA of the knee joint is an important one and has significant bearing in the field of total joint replacement and implant designs. The cause of the difference in patterns of joint wear is elusive, but genetic factors may be at work here.

■ Implants designed with the predominantly antero-medial degenerative patterns of knee joint wear of Caucasians in mind might not work as well if the pattern of wear is totally different.

■ This effect will even be magnified if the above point is not taken into account and one proceeds to a minimally invasive type of uni-compartmental knee replacement, which is very much in vogue nowadays.

References

1. Koskinen E, Paavolainen P, et al. (2007) Unicondylar knee replacement for primary osteoarthritis: A prospective follow-up study of 1,819 patients from the Finnish Arthroplasty Register. Acta Orthop, 78(1):128–35
2. Price AJ, Murray DW, et al. (2006) Simultaneous in vitro measurement of patellofemoral kinematics and forces following Oxford medial unicompartmental knee replacement. JBJS Br, 88(12):1591–5

Bisphosphonates and Peri-prosthetic Osteolysis

History and Examination

You saw a 75-year-old lady Jennifer, a retired painter and author, the other day in your orthopedic service. Jennifer had had a left total hip replacement done in another state 10 years ago, and had been found to have osteolysis around the implant near both the acetabular and femoral components on serial follow-up 2 years ago (Fig. 15). The attending surgeon decided to adopt a wait-and-see attitude and Jennifer was being prescribed daily bisphosphonate therapy plus calcium, even though the attending surgeon did not do a formal DXA scan. Jennifer had had a

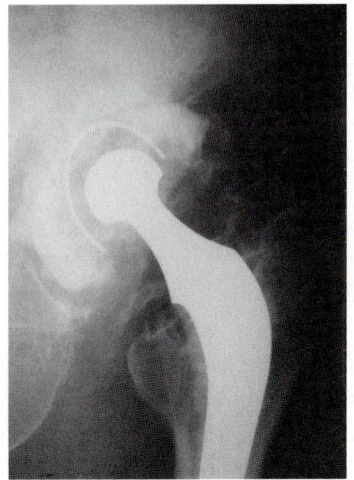

Fig. 15 Note the periprosthetic osteolysis from wear debris around the femoral and acetabular components of this total hip arthroplasty

fall 6 weeks earlier and was admitted to the same unit that performed the total hip replacement for her 10 years ago. The attending performed cerclage wiring for the peri-prosthetic fracture, and she was prescribed the "touch-down" type of weight-bearing exercise. A couple of weeks ago, Jennifer was visiting her mother in the state of California where you work. She felt increasing epigastric pain and heartburn and was admitted to the medical unit of your hospital. Gastroscopy revealed a large esophageal ulcer and bisphosphonates were stopped. The attending physician told Jennifer that he noticed incidentally peri-prosthetic bone loss or "osteolysis" around her left total hip. The physician then consulted you since Jennifer wishes to have a second opinion concerning her orthopedic problem and rehabilitation, wants to know more about the "osteolysis" that the physician has told her about, and whether bisphosphonates have really been doing her any good all along. Describe your opinion about the present case scenario and how would you manage or rehabilitate Jennifer's hip problem.

Discussion

The Swedish total joint registry has it that 80% of total joint failures are due to aseptic loosening and osteolysis. Aseptic loosening of total joint arthroplastics due to periprosthetic osteolysis is a frequent cause of implant failure, as in the present patient.

Different wear debris, particularly that of polyethylene, has been associated with periprosthetic osteolysis and loosening of total joint arthroplasties.

In normal bones, RANKL (receptor activator of NF-kappaB ligand), RANK (receptor activator of NF-kappaB) and OPG (osteoprotegerin) are three key molecules that regulate differentiation, survival, fusion, and activation of osteoclasts.

Wear debris primarily targets macrophages and osteoclast precursor cells, although osteoblasts, fibroblasts, and lymphocytes may also be involved as mentioned in the previous companion text to this book by the same author. The actual molecular responses include activation of

MAP kinase pathways, transcription factors including NFkappaB, and suppressors of cytokine signaling. This results in up-regulation of pro-inflammatory signaling and inhibition of the protective actions of anti-osteoclast cytokines such as interferon gamma.

Both polyethylene and other wear particles induce upregulation of RANK expression in cells of monocytic lineage, which may be important for periprosthetic osteoclastogenesis (Baumann et al., Acta Orthop Scand, 2004).

Considerable efforts are underway to develop therapies that identify novel targets for therapeutic intervention, in an attempt to tackle peri-prosthetic osteolysis around joint replacements.

In animal experiments in rats, the intra-articular injection of poly-ethylene particles caused substantial bone loss around a loaded implant. Alendronate was said to be effective in prevention and the particle-induced periprosthetic bone loss (Millett et al., JBJS, 2002).

Other support for the possible role of bisphosphonates (alendronate and zoledronate treatment) includes the increase in periprosthetic bone stock in a rabbit femoral model, particularly in the presence of UHM-WPE (ultra high molecular weight polyethylene) wear debris. These new findings suggest that bisphosphonates may more than compensate for the well-documented negative effects of wear debris on peri-implant bone stock (Von Knoch and Heckelei, J Biomed Mater Res A, 2005). In fact, there are recent studies even claiming the positive effect of bisphos-phonates, not only in the setting of implant-related osteolysis, but it is also claimed that it may enhance the process of osteo-integration of ti-tanium total joint implants in cementless fixation (Xing et al., J Biomed Mater Res, 2007).

However, other recent animal experiments at the University of Roch-ester Medical Center, New York, suggest that although bisphosphonates in adequate doses may cause apoptosis of osteoclasts (which is the main mechanism whereby bisphosphonates act as anti-resorptives in treating osteoporosis), but has little apparent effect on osteoclasts that are stimu-lated by inflammatory synovium pannus.

Scientists have thus considered other strategies like inhibition of the RANKL, which can cause apoptosis of such osteoclasts stimulated by inflammatory pannus to produce apoptosis, and thus may be even more effective in avoiding bony resorption.

On another front, studies from Harvard investigated the effect of exogenous OPG on ultra-high-molecular-weight polyethylene (UHM-WPE) particle-induced osteolysis. Exogenous OPG markedly suppressed UHMWPE particle-induced osteolysis in a murine calvarial model. This important finding underscores the crucial significance of the OPG-RANKL-RANK signaling in wear particle-induced osteolysis. Exogenous OPG may prove an effective treatment modality for wear debris-mediated periprosthetic osteolysis after total joint arthroplasty (Von Knoch and Heckelei, J Biomed Mater Res A, 2005).

Last, but not the least important, the new drug Denosumab (product of Amgen: The biggest world-wide bio-technology company, listed in Nasdaq) is a fully human monoclonal antibody that specifically targets the receptor activator of nuclear factor kappa B ligand (RANKL), a key mediator of the resorptive phase of bone remodeling. Denosumab is being studied across a whole range of conditions, including osteoporosis, treatment-induced bone loss, rheumatoid arthritis, bone metastases, and multiple myeloma. Whether it will have positive effects on peri-prosthetic osteolysis in the setting of aseptic loosening of total joint replacement remains to be seen.

Preliminary results with phase I and II clinical trials with AMG-162 (or Denosumab) have recently been completed. Based on these results AMG-162 appears to be safe and to have a potent effect on osteoclast function. Based on animal studies, it is expected that agents such as AMG-162 that block RANK-ligand/RANK interaction will have activity even in the setting of inflammation-induced osteolysis. Volumetric three-dimensional and MRI scans for detecting and quantifying peri-prosthetic osteolysis of the above-mentioned effect have been validated in cadaver studies and it will be very useful to document in future the drug's efficacy (Curr Opin Rheumatol).

Learning Point

- Despite promising results from animal experiments, there are as yet no approved treatments for osteolysis despite the promise of therapeutic agents against proinflammatory mediators (such as tumor necrosis factor) on osteoclasts shown in animal models (CORR, 2006). Use of bisphosphonates as a sole indication for peri-prosthetic implant-related bone loss instead of for osteoporosis seems to be too immature and needs to await proper randomised, double-blind placebo-controlled studies to prove its efficacy beyond an element of doubt. The surgeon who prescribed bisphosphonate for Jennifer might have used osteoporosis as the primary indication even though a formal DXA was not done.

- Currently, although supported by animal studies and isolated clinical case reports (O'Hara and Nivbrant, J Orthop Surg, 2004), the clinical efficacy of bisphosphonates in the context of managing peri-prosthetic osteolysis is not yet proven beyond doubt (Looney and Schwarz, Curr Opin Rheumatol, 2006).

- The use of exogenous OPG was found to be able to markedly suppress UHMWPE particle-induced osteolysis, and appears to be a promising agent.

References

1. Von Knoch F, Heckelei A (2005) Suppression of polyethylene particle-induced osteolysis by exogenous osteoprotegerin. J Biomed Mater Res A, 75(2):288–94
2. Looney RJ, Schwarz EM (2006) Periprosthetic osteolysis: An immunologist's update. Curr Opin Rheumatol, 18(1):80–7
3. Kinov P, Tivchev P, et al. (2006) Effect of risedronate on bone metabolism after total hip arthroplasty. Acta Orthop Belg, 72(1):44–50
4. O'Hara LJ, Nivbrant B (2004) Cross-linked polyethylene and bisphosphonate therapy for osteolysis in total hip arthroplasty: A case report. J Orthop Surg, 12(1):114–21
5. Talmo CT, Rubash HE, et al. (2006) Nonsurgical management of osteolysis: Challenges and opportunities. Clin Orthop Relat Res, 453:254–64

A Young Engineer with Disabling Sciatic Pain

History and Examination

You saw a new university graduate few months ago by the name of Harry, a mechanical engineer. Harry was lucky to find a job as a mechanical engineer after graduation and has frequently got to handle different machinery. Harry noticed acute right sciatic pain 6 weeks ago and had received physiotherapy for the same period in the form of McKenzie exercises, traction, interferential therapy, and short-wave diathermy with only mild improvement. There was no neurological deficit. The MRI report showed a moderate-sized postero-lateral disc prolapse without accompanying Modic changes. Harry now seeks your help as a rehabilitation specialist, but he told you in advance that he would prefer not to have an operation if possible, although he would like to know the pros and cons of different options. How would you proceed to manage and counsel Harry?

Discussion

You started by telling Harry about the functional components of the normal intervertebral disc: Which consists of:

- The nucleus pulposus with high water and proteoglycans
- Inner annulus, a structure that resembles fibrocartilage, more type 2 than 1 collagen
- Outer annulus, more type 1 than 2 collagen, resists tensile strain and disc bulge
- End plate, resembles hyaline cartilage, deforms on compression, and with porosity to allow diffusion across to the relative avascular disc

The normal disc functions to support high compressive loads, up to a few times the body weight from muscle action, as well as support high tensile loads by the annulus, while maintaining stability and flexibility of the spine. In general, it is the degenerate disc, not the aged disc, that is prone to herniation, sometimes triggered by trauma creating a tear of the annulus. Aging alone will not decrease the disc space to any significant extent; however, loss of disc space on X-ray is seen with a degraded or degenerate disc. Thus, some special triggers are likely required to commence the process of disc degeneration. Likely triggers include possible end-plate rupture and/or an auto-immune process that resembles that of sympathetic ophthalmia. Most recently, the role of genetic factors in controlling the relative proportion of collagen in the disc has been implicated. You further told Harry that most cases of postero-lateral disc prolapse can be managed conservatively. Even for those cases in which operation is needed for simple herniation, the results after operation, although better at 1 year, the end result at 3–5 years is about the same.

McKenzie exercises

These back exercises are named after a physical therapist in New Zealand who found that extending the spine through exercise could reduce pain generated from a compromised disc space. Theoretically, extension exercises may also help reduce the herniation of the disc itself and reduce pressure on a nerve root. There is in fact a wide range of McKenzie exercises, some of which are done standing up, while others are performed lying down. All of them use core muscle contraction and usually arm motions as well to stabilize the trunk and extend the spine.

For patients who are suffering from leg pain due to a disc herniation as in Harry's case, extending the spine with McKenzie back exercises may also help reduce the leg pain by "centralizing" the pain, i.e., moving the pain from the leg to the back. For most patients, back pain is usually more tolerable than leg pain, and if a patient is able to centralize the pain, they may be able to continue with non-surgical treatment and may ultimately avoid a surgical discectomy. When the pain is acute, the exercises should be done frequently (every 1–2 h). To be effective, patients should try to avoid flexing the spine (bending forward) during exercising as this undercuts the strengthening motion. In the present case scenario, McKenzie exercises did meet with some partial initial success in allaying Harry's symptomatology.

Traction

The current evidence suggests that traction is probably not uniformly effective and it did not work for our patient Harry. A recent Cochrane Review commented that neither continuous nor intermittent traction by itself was more effective in improving pain, disability or work absence than placebo, sham or other treatments for patients with a mixed duration of lower back pain, with or without sciatica (Clarke et al., Cochrane Database Syst Rev, 2005).

FIRST II Trial (Finnish Infliximab-related Study)

In recent years, tumor necrosis factor alpha (TNF-α) has been established as an important mediator in intervertebral disc herniation-induced sciatica in animal models. Early open-label studies, i.e., studies with a concurrent control treatment, suggested that anti-TNF-α treatment was potentially effective for the treatment of sciatica. The results of initial uncontrolled studies from Finland showed the beneficial effect of a single infusion of infliximab 3 mg/kg for herniation-induced sciatica over a 1-year follow-up period.

However, in a recent, properly designed randomized controlled trial known as the FIRST II (Finnish Infliximab Related Study), designed for investigating patients with unilateral sciatic pain associated with a disc herniation with concordant symptoms and signs of radicular pain; the trial demonstrated no difference in efficacy between infliximab, versus placebo. The authors of the trial concluded that although the long-term results of this randomized trial do not support the use of infliximab compared with placebo for lumbar radicular pain in patients with disc herniation-induced sciatica, further study in a subgroup of patients with L4–L5 or L3–L4 herniations, especially in the presence of Modic changes, appears to be warranted (Spine, 2006). The obvious next question that Harry asked about at this juncture centers on "MRI Modic Changes".

Modic Changes

Another recent study in Finland investigates the possible associations of frequency and intensity of LBP and sciatic pain with Modic changes in a sample of middle-aged male workers with or without whole-body vibration exposure at work. It was found that 80% of MRI Modic changes occurred at L4–L5 or L5–S1. Modic changes at L5–S1 showed significant association with pain symptoms with increased frequency of LBP (odds ratio 2.28; 95% confidence interval 1.44–3.15) and sciatica episodes (odds ratio 1.44; 95% confidence interval 1.01–1.89), and with higher LBP visual analog scores Modic changes at L5–S1 and Modic type I lesions are more likely to be associated with pain symptoms than other types of Modic changes or changes located at other lumbar levels. In Harry's case, the radiologist did not notice Modic changes on his MRI.

Overall Comments on Conservative Treatment

A recent systematic review in 2007 assesses as many as 30 trials that included injections, traction, physical therapy, bed rest, manipulation, medication, and acupuncture as treatment for the lumbosacral sciatica. The authors commented that whether clinicians should prescribe physical therapy, bed rest, manipulation or medication could not be concluded from the review as not one of them stands alone as being definitely superior (Luijsterburg et al., Eur Spine J, 2007). Before we explore the efficacy of surgery, Harry asked about steroid injections via the epidural or transforaminal route?

Epidural Injection

Although an epidural injection can usually provide quick and significant pain relief in sciatica, the action is usually short, lasting around 2–3 months and has to be repeated.

Although its routine use is being questioned by many (JAMA, 2007), there are situations where epidural or transforaminal steroids do work and relieve the patient of suffering, particularly if the patient declines surgical intervention (Young et al., J Am Acad Orthop Surg, 2007). Personally, the author is in favor of the transforaminal route (Fig. 16) and this was the modality that finally relieved Harry's pain. At the time of

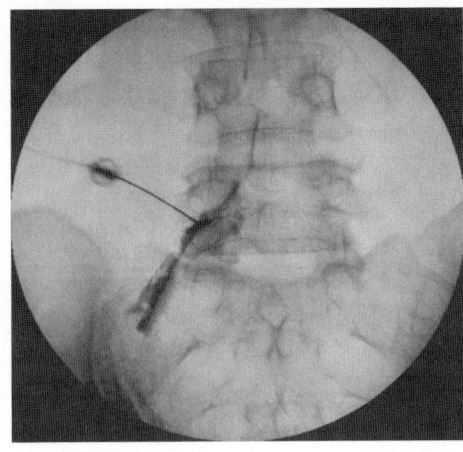

Fig. 16 Radiograph showing the epidural steroid injection under fluoroscopic guidance

writing of this book, Harry remained pain free 1 year after the transforaminal injection, and was put on maintenance hydrotherapy.

Surgery

Disc prolapse accounts for 5% of lower back disorders, but is one of the most common reasons for surgery. Only four trials have directly compared discectomy with conservative management and these trials gave suggestive rather than conclusive results, although there is suggestion that discectomy produces better clinical outcomes than chemonucleolysis and that in turn is better than placebo. Microdiscectomy gives broadly comparable results to standard discectomy. Recent trials of an inter-position gel covering the dura (five trials) and of fat (four trials) showed that they can reduce scar formation, although there is limited evidence of the effect on clinical outcomes. There is insufficient evidence on other percutaneous discectomy techniques to draw firm conclusions from these. Three small randomized control trial (RCTs) of laser discectomy do not again provide conclusive evidence of their efficacy. There are no published RCTs of coblation therapy or trans-foraminal endoscopic discectomy.

In a recent *Cochrane Review* in 2007, the authors found that surgical discectomy for carefully selected patients with sciatica due to lumbar disc prolapse may provide faster relief from the acute attack than conservative management, although any positive or negative effects on the lifetime natural history of the underlying disc disease are still unclear. Microdiscectomy tends to give broadly comparable results to open discectomy. The evidence on other minimally invasive techniques still remains unclear (Gibson and Waddell, Cochrane Database Syst Rev, 2007).

Comparing Effects of Early Vs. Late Surgery

An article looking at this aspect appeared in the May 2007 issue of NEJM, in which 283 patients who had had severe sciatica for 6–12 weeks were randomly assigned to have early surgery or to prolonged conservative treatment with surgery if needed. The primary outcomes were the score on the Roland Disability Questionnaire, the score on the visual analogue scale for leg pain, and the patient's report of perceived recovery during the first year after randomization.

It was found that although the 1-year outcomes were similar for patients assigned to early surgery and those assigned to conservative treatment with eventual surgery if needed, the rates of pain relief and of perceived recovery were faster for those assigned to early surgery (Peul et al., N Engl J Med, 2007).

Learning Point

- Although compression of a nerve root does not always cause pain, pain is the rule if the nerve root is inflamed.
- It is believed that not uncommonly, chemical irritants like Substance P, PG, etc., from the disc may be the cause of the chemical irritation causing root inflammation.
- That is why there has recently been an enthusiasm for special drug treatments like infliximab, which has been studied in large clinical trials in the Finnish Infliximab-Related Study.

- For patients refractory to conventional physical therapy and who refuse surgery, there may be a place for either epidural or transforaminal steroids, and the author favours the latter among patients reluctant to have surgery.
- Although previous natural history studies on lumbar disc prolapse-related sciatica tend to show comparable outcome at the 2-year mark, the recent Cochrane reviews tend to re-confirm that surgery is instrumental in providing more speedy recovery and better short-term outcome.
- Patients who are undecided about the different treatment options should thus be properly counselled and briefed on the latest clinical findings.

References

1. Timo Korhonen, et al. (2006) The treatment of disc-herniation-induced sciatica with infliximab: One-year follow-up results of FIRST II, a randomized controlled trial, Spine, 31(24):2759–66

2. Gibson J, Waddell G (2007) Surgical interventions for lumbar disc prolapse, Cochrane Database Syst Rev, 18 (2):CD001350

3. Clarke JA, van Tulder MW. et al. (2005) Traction for low-back pain with or without sciatica. Cochrane Database Syst Rev, (4):CD003010

4. Kuisma M, Karppinen J, et al. (2007) Modic changes in endplates of lumbar vertebral bodies: Prevalence and association with low back and sciatic pain among middle-aged male workers. Spine, 32(10):1116–22

5. Hampton T (2007) Epidurals' benefit for back pain questioned. JAMA, 297(16):1757–8

6. Young IA, Hyman GS, et al. (2007) The use of lumbar epidural/transforaminal steroids for managing spinal disease. J Am Acad Orthop Surg, 15(4):228–38

7. Luijsterburg PA, Verhagen AP, et al. (2007) Effectiveness of conservative treatments for the lumbosacral radicular syndrome: A systematic review. Eur Spine J, 16(7):881–99

8. Peul WC, van Houwelingen HC, et al. (2007) Surgery vs prolonged conservative treatment for sciatica. N Engl J Med, 356:2245–56

9. www.remicade.com (web source for the drug infliximab)

The "Wonder Drug" Glucosamine

History and Examination

You saw 63-year-old Mrs Gibbons the other day in your orthopedic clinic, a retired shop-keeper with mainly right knee pain for the past 3 years. Mrs Gibbons was seen all this time by her family physician, who diagnosed right knee osteoarthritis as well as early osteoarthritis on the left side. Her family physician treated Mrs Gibbons with various trials of non-steroidal anti-inflammatory agents, on and off short courses of physiotherapy, but to no avail. He introduced the drug glucosamine to Mrs Gibbons 12 months ago and told Mrs Gibbons that she can consider long-term glucosamine for her knee problem. But when Mrs Gibbons chatted with her friends with similar knee problems, some of them told her that their doctors told them there is no concrete evidence that this drug needs to be taken indefinitely. Feeling rather perplexed, Mrs Gibbons asked for an orthopedic opinion and went to see you. On examination, Mrs Gibbons proved to be an obese lady weighing 85 kg, with relatively normal tibio-femoral alignment although Mrs Gibbons does walk with an adduction moment. There was also minimal knee effusion on the right side. There was mild right knee quadriceps weakness, with bilateral crepitus and the motion of the right knee was 15–120°, although it was full on the left side. Review of the radiographs showed early medial compartment osteoarthritis on the left side, and marked antero-medial compartment osteoarthritis quite typical of the pattern we expect for Caucasians. Describe what will be your subsequent management of Mrs Gibbons as well as your evidence-based advice concerning the drug glucosamine – the main reason Mrs Gibbons came to you.

Discussion

Glucosamine is a natural amino sugar and a normal constituent of glycosaminoglycans in the cartilage matrix and synovial fluid of joints. Crystalline glucosamine sulfate salt has been approved as a medicinal product for the treatment of osteoarthritis in several European countries.

Although it has been prescribed for more than 10 years, it is only due to the research in the last few years that the scientific bases underlying its beneficial effects are starting to unveil. Given at the oral dosage of 1,500 mg per day, it is popular among family physicians in treating patients with knee OA symptoms like Mrs Gibbons.

Despite its popularity, as pointed out by a recent Cochrane systematic review, not all trials have found it to have a definite positive effect on the symptomatic control of osteo-arthrotic knee.

Examples of studies in favor of glucosamine include a recent randomized, double-blind, placebo-controlled trial in which this compound allegedly could clinically control pain and produce beneficial effects in patients with knee osteoarthritis, with the authors claiming the drug may possibly delay the appearance of long-term structural changes in the joint. Whether these claims are borne out in practice depends on long-term follow-up studies. But the fact that it has an excellent toxicity profile scores positively for this product. The findings of a recent study suggested that glucosamine sulfate at the oral daily dosage of 1,500 mg is more effective than placebo in treating knee OA symptoms. Although acetaminophen also had a higher responder rate compared with placebo, it failed to show significant effects on the algofunctional indexes (Herreo-Beaumont et al., Arthritis Rheum, 2007).

Currently, the mechanism of action of glucosamine sulfate still remains to be clearly elucidated. However, the activity of glucosamine sulfate has recently been related to its possible capacity to down-regulate the catabolic effects of pro-inflammatory molecules, such as IL-1, which are present in osteoarthritic cartilage (Herreo-Beaumont et al., Expert Opin Pharmacother, 2007). Other studies revealed possible inhibition of aggrecanese-mediated loss of GAG, possibly via a possible anti-inflammatory effect via action on the production of TNF-α, IL-1β, and PGE2 in macrophages (Kim et al., Bioorg Med Chem Lett, 2007).

On the other hand, some trials like that conducted by Baime and co-workers did *not* show a clinical response (Evid Based Med, 2006); while some other workers also cast uncertainties on the usefulness of "supplements" for arthritis (Hampton, JAMA, 2007). Another challenge as regards oral glucosamine sulphate is that despite claims that it might increase glycosaminoglycan (GAG) synthesis in chondrocytes, the low level of the substance achieved in the synovial fluid after the *oral* route might not be adequate for GAG synthesis. This phenomenon seems to be borne out by animal studies in bovines recently.

Evaluation of whether patient characteristics and/or radiographic disease patterns predict symptomatic response to treatment with glucosamine in knee osteoarthritis is of practical importance and was reported in a recent study in the British Journal of Sports Medicine. In this study, glucosamine may be more effective at improving symptoms in knee OA patients with a lower body mass index, PFJ osteophytes and lower functional self-efficacy (Bennett et al., Br J Sports Med, 2007).

Subsequent Patient Management

After provision of the current clinical knowledge of the drug glucosamine, Mrs Gibbons was satisfied and decided to stop the drug as she had taken the medication for more than 12 months with mediocre effect. She followed your advice and attended weight loss classes run by your hospital's dietician, participated in physiotherapy to re-train her weakened quadriceps in addition to pain relief modalities. You subsequently performed a gait analysis and the kinetics report confirmed a significant right knee adduction moment. She was given an anti-knee adduction moment knee brace from Donjoy, which relieves her pain while walking. She managed to lose 8 kg of weight, and later participated in hydrotherapy classes that you prescribed her including under-water walking exercises. She was finally put on maintenance Tai-Chi exercise after all the above treatment courses were finished to re-train her knee joint proprioception and postural stability.

Learning Point

- Several non-pharmacological therapies such as exercise, education and weight loss can have an effect on patients with knee pain, though the effect was reported to be modest in the literature. Ultrasound and short-wave diathermy are widely available, but not much supported by evidence according to a recent Cochrane Systematic Review.
- Glucosamine is popular, but not all trials have found it to have any effect. Non-steroidal anti-inflammatory drugs (NSAIDs) have a modest effect and their long-term value has not yet been established. They are associated with significant adverse events, particularly gastrointestinal haemorrhage, which has a substantial risk of mortality. They are particularly dangerous in the elderly.
- Every once in a while, we do see ladies with mainly medial OA knee pain walking with a significant adduction moment. This can sometimes be helped by an anti-adduction moment knee brace during gait as in this case scenario. Weight loss is likely to help in providing pain relief on negotiating stairs, particularly for patients with patello-femoral joint (PFJ) OA of the knee as the PFJ forces on walking stairs will be much reduced after weight loss.
- A brand new armamentarium in the conservative treatment of symptomatic knee OA is acupuncture. That it may represent a potentially valuable treatment for OA knee, and the evidence on effectiveness, safety and cost was looked into recently and it is awaiting further research (White, Acupuncture Med, 2006).

References

1. Bliddal H, et al. (2006) Glucosamine effectiveness in the treatment of knee osteoarthritis. Presentation of a Cochrane analysis with the perspective on the GAIT trial, Ugeskr Laeger, 168(50):4405–9

2. Baime MJ, et al. (2006) Glucosamine and chondroitin sulphate did not improve pain in osteoarthritis of the knee,Evid Based Med, 11(4):115

3. Herreo-Beaumont G, Ivorra JA, et al. (2007) Glucosamine sulphate in the treatment of knee arthritis symptoms: A randomized double-blind, placebo-controlled study using acetaminophen as a side comparator. Arthritis Rheum, 56(2):555–67

4. Kim MM, Mendis E, et al. (2007) Glucosamine sulphate promotes osteoblastic differentiation of MG-63 cells via anti-inflammatory effect. Bioorg Med Chem Lett, 17(7):1938–42

5. Hampton T (2007) Efficacy still uncertain for widely used supplements for arthritis. JAMA, 297(4):351–2

6. Bennett AN, Crossley KM, et al. (2007) Predictors of symptomatic response to glucosamine in knee osteoarthritis: An exploratory study. Br J Sports Med, 41(7):415–9

7. Pollo FE, Jackson RW (2006) Knee bracing for unicompartmental osteoarthritis. J Am Acad Orthop Surg, 14(1):5–11

Hyaluronan for Knee OA, Facts Vs. Myths

History and Examination

You saw Mrs Simmons, who is a 70-year-old retired librarian, the other day in your clinic as a new case. It transpires that Mrs Simmons has a history of bilateral tricompartmental knee osteoarthritis, managed all along by her family doctor, who prescribed on and off physiotherapy, and now strongly advises that Mrs Simmons should receive periodic injection of the drug hyaluronan to "prevent the joint from deteriorating". Mrs Simmons does not feel much difference after a few injections, but found that the treatment is very expensive as she has no income after her retirement. She now requests to see a rehabilitation specialist like you for your opinion on this drug. How would you proceed?

Discussion

Although intra-articular injections of steroids are not infrequently used by many primary care physicians in tackling significant OA knee symptoms and may be effective at least if only for a short period; intra-articular hyaluronan has a longer duration of action and in general tends to be safer. Patients in general prefer treatments that are safe. This is particularly so in the subgroup of patients of OA knee patients with active synovitis wherein intra-articular steroids can potentially cause systemic side effects, especially if the patient happens to have multiple concomitant medical co-morbidities, which is not uncommon, such as resulting in causing fluid retention in a patient with pre-existing cardiac or renal disease. Another sub-group of patients in which the author will absolutely avoid steroids includes those who are immunocompromised or infection-prone, as well as those with significant diminished joint position sense and peripheral neuropathy, particularly if concomitant malalignment of lower limb mechanical axis is present.

Hyaluronan is one of the major space-filling molecules in the extracellular matrix of the articular cartilage, which has a visco-elastic function to help protect the joint from periodic loading. Thanks to the works of scientists like Vincent Hascall in Cleveland, Ohio, we now know more about the mechanism of the origin of the visco-elasticity. Hyaluronan is in fact organized into the extracellular matrix by specific interactions with other matrix macromolecules. However, high molecular weight hyaluronan at a high concentration in solution can also form entangled molecular networks through steric interactions and self-association between and within individual molecules. The latter configuration can occur when a stretch of the hydrophobic face of the ribbon structure of the backbone interacts reversibly with the hydrophobic face on a comparable stretch of hyaluronan on another molecule or in a different region of the same molecule. Such networks exhibit different properties than isolated hyaluronan molecules. They can resist rapid, short-duration fluid flow through the network, thereby exhibiting elastic properties that can distribute load or shear forces within the network. This kind of structure is ideally suited to the dynamic periodic peak joint loading conditions to which our knee is subjected during normal gait.

The first medical application of hyaluronan for humans was as a vitreous supplement/replacement during eye surgery in the late 1950s. The hyaluronan used was isolated initially from human umbilical cord, and shortly thereafter from rooster combs in a highly purified and high molecular weight form. This latter preparation is now sold under the trade name of Healon. Another hyaluronan product, Artz, was developed for use as a supplement in the synovium of osteoarthritic joints, and a covalently cross-linked form of hyaluronan, Synvisc (Biomatrix), with more pronounced viscoelastic properties, is also being used for the same purpose.

It is the author's view that hyaluronan is currently being mainly used for their possible visco-supplementation effect rather than having objective evidence-based support for being directly beneficial in other settings like acute cartilage injury or tears, although the occasional expert in chondral repair does add hyaluronan after arthroscopic chondroplasty to their patients. Similarly, there is paucity of scientific evidence of a direct action of hyaluronan on the degenerate articular surface of arthritic joints.

Conclusion

Given the current evidence, there are still reservations regarding the routine use of intra-articular hyaluronan in knee arthritis, as there are still uncertainties on the usefulness of many "supplements" for arthritis, as also pointed out by Hampton in JAMA, 2007.

Learning Point

- Hyaluronan is currently being mainly used for its possible visco-supplementation effect rather than having objective evidence-based support for being directly beneficial in other settings like acute cartilage injury or tears although the occasional expert in chondral repair does administer hyaluronan to their patients after arthroscopic chondroplasty.
- Patients should be made aware of the current understanding of the agent, and the transient nature of whatever benefit (if any) therefrom, before actually spending large amounts of money on the agent.

References

1. Laurent TC (ed) (1998) The chemistry, biology and medical applications of hyaluronan and its derivatives. Wenner-Gren International Series, vol 72, Portland Press, London
2. Hampton T (2007) Efficacy still uncertain for widely used supplements for arthritis. JAMA, 297(4):351–2

History and Examination

You received a referral from a physician the other day concerning a middle-aged lady with bilateral forefoot pain, Mrs Jennings. She turns out to be the senior administrative executive of a famous local bank. It transpires that Mrs Jennings has history of bilateral forefoot pain especially at the base of the second toes of both feet, which she noted has developed local skin thickenings on the plantar surface. Mrs Jennings also noticed that both her second toes are now deformed and that the pain gets worse when she wears her high heels for work. In fact, Mrs Jennings has had the habit of wearing high-heeled shoes for the past 8–10 years as she thinks they look nice and make her seemed taller. However, for the past 1 year, she has been noticing increasing leg cramps in both her calves as well as pre-tibial muscles. In one instance, the leg cramps and pain in the second toes got so suddenly painful while she attempted to chase a bus going to work that she tripped over and fell, with abrasions on both her forearms and knee caps.

On examination, the lower limb tibio-femoral alignment appear satisfactory; there was no muscle wasting. Obvious callosities had developed at the second metatarsal heads of both feet with bilateral hammer toes. There was no significant pes planus nor pes cavus, the heel alignment appeared normal.

Further examination revealed that both her triceps surae were tight and her hamstrings were also tight and had some pain on stretching. Luckily, both the hammer toes were still flexible, and there was not (yet) any significant degree of hallux valgus. Do you think that chronic wearing of high-heeled shoe-wear may have contributed to her forefoot problems and muscle spasms? If so, what is the pathogenesis and how would you manage your patient?

Discussion

In order to understand the effect of chronic wearing of high heels on the human gait, one has to first understand the function of various muscle groups in normal gait discussed in detail in the companion textbook by the same author, but some key points are again highlighted here, viz.:

- The triceps surae muscle group plays a key role in human gait as its action is involved in *all* the three key rockers as previously described by Perry and others. Essentially, there is eccentric contraction of this muscle group during the first and second rockers and concentric contraction during the third rocker. During the first rocker, there is controlled plantarflexion of the ankle to aid in shock absorption and prevent the landing foot from slapping onto the ground. During the second rocker, eccentric contraction of this muscle group aids in the smooth anterior translation of the tibia over the stationary foot, while during the third rocker, concentric contraction of the triceps surae provides the power for push-off and act as the so-called "power house" of human gait.

- In normal gait, the mechanism to counteract the knee joint of the landing leg to buckle depends very much on controlled plantarflexion, so as to effect the so-called plantarflexion-knee extension couple, i.e., providing an external extension knee moment in order to stabilize the knee; thus, if this controlled plantar-flexion is affected by whatever cause, the person will need to use much higher quadriceps force to counteract the diminished or even absent extension knee moment.

- In normal gait, the ankle dorsiflexors effect eccentric contraction for smooth loading, while concentric contraction occurs to ensure proper foot clearance in swing.

- Other decelerators and "brakes" include the hip extensors (hamstrings and/or gluteus maximus) that are active in terminal swing and the loading response.

- Finally, smoothness in swing requires the action of hip flexors or iliopsoas and proper muscle control and relaxation of the quadriceps around the knee.

Clinical Implications

- The wearing of high heels has the potential to decrease the efficiency of shock absorption since *all* the three rockers as described by Perry will be affected. The negative effect on the smooth functioning of the three rockers will diminish shock absorption and increase the impact forces on the whole kinetic chain as well as on the spine.
- Most chronic wearers of high heels end up, therefore, with variable tightness of the triceps surae muscle group and tendo-achilles.
- A triceps surae that is chronically tight and and/or shortened, may weaken the push-off action during toe-off at terminal stance.
- If the wearing of high heels is coupled with the wearing of shoes with a narrow toe box, this may predispose to hammer toes and/or hallux valgus with chronic wear.
- There is also an increased chance of or predisposition to sprained ankle as the contact point of the heel on the ground is much diminished.

Other Gait Laboratory Findings for High Heels

In a recent gait laboratory study, five young women in their 20s wore 7-cm tall high-heeled shoes vs. sneakers, and walked in a 10-m gait laboratory walkway. Inverse dynamics was used to analyze the torques at the ankle, knee and hip. Results showed that peak adduction moments at the knee and ankle increased and flexion/extension moments at the hip increased with high-heeled shoes compared with the sneakers. The high-heeled shoes resulted in a greater load in the lower limb joints, especially to the knee and hip (Hao et al., Conf Proc IEEE Eng Med Biol Soc, 2005).

Functional Consequence of High Heels

In effect, the metatarsal heads then become the main pivot point instead of the ankle after wearing high-heeled shoes. Force concentration on the forefoot will be higher the higher the heel height.

Tibial advance blocked in the second rocker is affected by an artificially induced forced equines posture, the trunk tends to flex forwards to keep the center of the mass over the base of support.

Swing requires increased hip flexion for foot clearance. Those with weak calf muscles tend to take shorter steps in order to keep the weight from getting too far ahead of the ankle, and more quadriceps activation (thus easier to fatigue) is needed to keep the knee from buckling and hold the tibia back.

Management

- Treatment frequently includes tendo-archilles stretching since it is usually tight; for more severe cases I prescribe a night-time AFO (ankle foot arthrosis). Those with weak triceps surae need to train up the pre-tibial muscles. Management of hammer toes is along the guidelines described in the companion texts by the same author. Measuring and documenting the abnormal distribution of foot pressure by Tekscan is useful (Figs. 17, 18).

- Although most clinicians advise avoidance of further wear of high heels, there are two groups of ladies in whom this advice may not be useful The first group include those whose job nature mandates

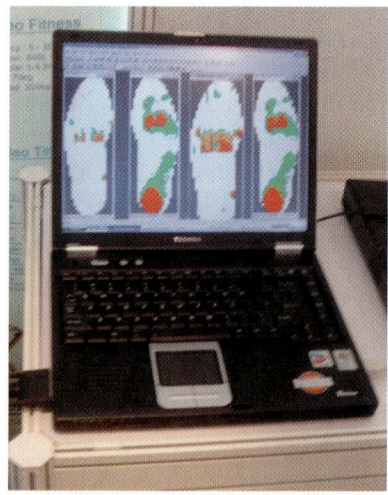

Fig. 17 Commercially available Tekscan to assess distribution of plantar pressures

them to wear high heels and who do not intend to quit or change their job; the second group are those ladies who believe that the wearing of high heels is so essential to their general appearance that anything else is of only secondary importance. So, the question is how to tackle these two groups of patients? One possible answer probably lies in the findings of research on gait analysis as described in the section that follows.

Further Biomechanics Data from Gait Analysis

An interesting recent gait and biomechanics study showed that in persons wearing high heels, the plantar pressure in the heel and mid-foot shifted to the medial forefoot, and the vertical and anteroposterior GRF increased. Use of the TCI (total contact inserts) reduces the peak pressure in the medial forefoot. Interestingly, the effectiveness of the TCI was greater in the users of higher heels than in those with lower heels and flat heels. The peak pressure in the medial forefoot, impact force, and the first peak vertical GRF could explain 75.6% of the variance of comfort in high-heeled gait. The authors concluded that wearing high heels results in decreased comfort, which can be reflected by both the subjective rating scale and biomechanical variables. Use of a TCI shoe

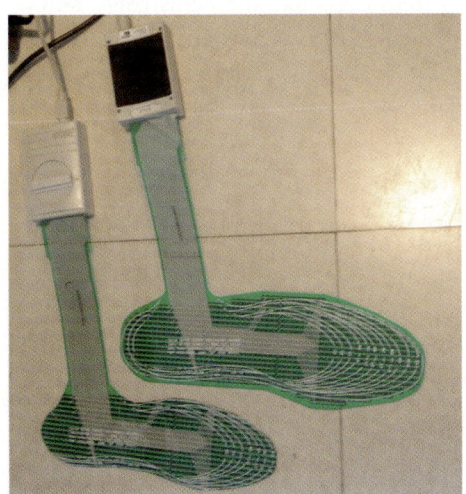

Fig. 18 Close-up of the pressure sensors of the Tekscan feeding signals to the computer

insert alters the biomechanics and therefore may improve the comfort in wearers of high-heeled shoes (Hong et al., Foot Ankle Int, 2005).

Learning Point

- The disadvantages of chronic use of high heels is well known to orthopedic surgeons and to most primary care physicians. However, most orthopods and family physicians usually just give the general advice to patients of avoiding high-heeled shoes and doing some stretching. However, to face reality, some ladies do work in companies that require their lady staff to wear high heels. To advise this important subgroup of patients as well as those lady patients who refuse to forsake their high heels just to give up high heels is not really very realistic.

- In these cases, a combination of total contact shoe insert, wearing proper-sized shoes with a wider shoe box, stretching of tight triceps surae, and considering using special types of rocker-bottom athletic shoes during weekends and off work (see Fig. 19) is advised. The rocker-bottom type of registered trademark MBT shoe wear was found by the author to have the advantage of re-training the idle and less used leg muscles with chronic wearing of high heels like the hamstrings, and the triceps surae; besides it also helps re-train the proprioceptive sense of the ankle joint (Ip, submitted for publication).

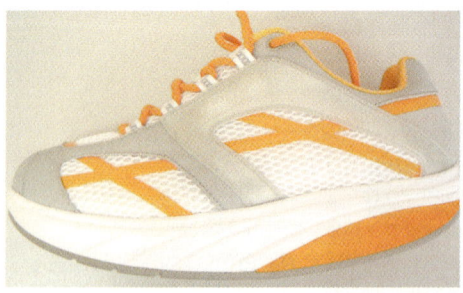

Fig. 19 Notice the rocker-bottom of this type of athletic shoes marketed under the trade name MBT

References

1. Hao Z, Zhou J, et al. (2005) Different plantar interface effects on dynamics of the lower limb Conf Proc IEEE Eng Med Biol Soc, 6:6021–4
2. Hong WH, Lee YH, et al. (2005) Influence of heel height and shoe insert on comfort perception and biomechanical performance of young female adults during walking. Foot Ankle Int, 26(12):1042–8

Silent Bone Loss and Vitamin D Insufficiency

History and Examination

Francis is a 67-year-old retired high school teacher living in Utah. She suffered from a left Colles' fracture 2 years ago after losing balance in the supermarket. She went to see a government hospital where casting was done. She was given calcium and vitamin D besides physiotherapy on clinic follow-up when the cast was taken off. However, during the next clinic follow-up, another young orthopedic surgeon took her off the calcium and vitamin D, did a radiograph of her left wrist, told her that the bone looked fine and that there was no need for follow-up. Since the fall, Francis has been going out very infrequently as she is afraid of falling again. This was made worse by the fact that she was widowed last year with her husband dying of a cerebrovascular event, and she has no children. One year ago, she had another fall in the wet bathroom and sustained a 20% wedge compression fracture of her L1 vertebral body. She was treated by the same young orthopedic surgeon who closed her file last year when she was admitted to the orthopedic unit.

The young surgeon asked Francis to leave the hospital after staying for 3 days and wrote a referral to the physiotherapy department. Francis requested the young surgeon to check for osteoporosis, but was declined. She left the hospital in misery with a handful of pain-killers, a physiotherapy referral, and a clinic appointment 3 months later. Francis used her precious money to see a private orthopod who ordered a DXA scan. The T-score was found to be −2.8 and the private orthopod prescribed risedronate for Francis. Francis had good compliance with her medication but has a further fear of going outdoors; she orders her daily essentials either over the phone or via the internet. Six weeks ago amid the winter snow, Francis had a fall in her doorway while clearing some snow from the front door, and was admitted to your orthopedic unit for fractured neck of the femur at the left hip. You asked the hospital's endocrinologist to do a 1,25 di(OH) vitamin D assay and it turned out to be nearly undetectable, even on double checking. In this case scenario, do you think vitamin D deficiency could have predisposed Francis to multiple fractures? Describe your further management of Francis.

Discussion

General Introduction

The great importance of ensuring replete calcium and vitamin D among our patient population with fragility fractures in particular has not been stressed enough in many standard orthopedic textbooks in the past. It is high time that orthopedic surgeons reminded themselves of this important information faced with an aging population and soaring number of fragility fractures. The importance lies in the fact that calcium and vitamin D intake modulate age-related increases in the PTH levels of bone resorption and occult PTH increases do in fact contribute to the pathogenesis of osteoporosis and lessen the effects of whatever expensive anti-osteoporosis medications our patients may be taking.

Sub-clinical vitamin D deficiency and secondary hyperparathyroidism is very common in patients with osteoporosis, but this fact is very often underestimated (Utiger, N Engl J Med, 1998).

Epidemiology for Calcium and Vitamin D

Current WHO guidelines on "Consultation on Mineral Requirements in Human Nutrition" made it clear that the recommendations for calcium intake were based on long-term calcium balance data for adults derived from Australia, Canada, the European Union, the United Kingdom and the United States, and not necessarily applicable to all countries worldwide. The report acknowledged that strong evidence was emerging that the requirements for calcium might vary from culture to culture for dietary, genetic, lifestyle and geographical reasons. On this score, the said committee did mention that one should avoid excess intake of animal protein in the diet lest there is interference with calcium absorption – thus solving the so-called "calcium paradox" that describes a seemingly higher incidence of fragility fractures in populations with a high intake of calcium-rich dairy products. The international recommendation nowadays of calcium intake is at least 1,200 mg per day. For the elderly, especially those living alone and in institutions like nursing homes in particular, calcium supplementation is highly recommended. At the same time as avoiding excess animal protein, other foods rich in calcium can be considered for the elderly, such as fresh green vegetables, tofu, cheese, etc., although these choices are of course suitable for the general population as well. Thus, excessive intake of daily products (with lots of acidic animal proteins) might outweigh the positive effect of calcium intake on calcium balance as a whole.

Studies in the USA indicate that only about 50% of the adult population is meeting its calcium and D needs, and it has been estimated that over 80% vitamin D deficiency is reported in a hospitalized fracture population. The minimal healthy vitamin D serum level is at least 30 ng/ml. If less than 30, parameters of secondary hyperparathyroidism are usually present and contribute to the development of osteoporosis. More recent recommendations by workers like Holic and others advise a level between 35 and 55 ng/ml, instead of the traditional figure of 30 ng/ml.

Importance of Calcium and Vitamin D

It is common knowledge that the serum calcium level of humans has to be maintained within narrow limits, especially for neuromuscular tissues, and a multitude of other cellular functions, including enzymes. Our body's store of calcium is found mainly in our skeleton as hydroxyapatite crystals. Our body's in-built homeostasis system is such that the above-mentioned calcium level in the circulation is properly maintained, even at the expense of resorption of the skeleton if and whenever the need arises.

Vitamin D plays an important role in the regulation of calcium levels as well as bone mineralisation, among many other functions, and in fact vitamin D is now regarded as a hormone. Its deficiency causes osteomalacia or rickets, while its insufficiency can exacerbate osteoporosis. Other important roles include gait balance strength particularly in the elderly, and its effect on the immune system. In addition, the Framingham Study revealed that low intake and low serum levels of vitamin D are in fact associated with increased risk of OA progression.

An interesting recent basic science study from the University of Toronto based on the use of the well-known MNX guinea pig model of severe OA revealed that vitamin D can affect the progression of OA, but not the onset of OA. In fact, a lack of vitamin D together with OA can potentiate cartilage degradation, since OA bone appears to be more sensitive to changes in vitamin D levels compared with normal bone (ORS Proceedings, 2007).

Calcium/Vitamin D and Fracture Risk Reduction

Calcium supplementation and vitamin D slows loss of BMD, decreases bone turnover over 4 years, and reduces fracture incidence in elderly adults. It is a cost-effective weak antiresorptive and can decrease hip fractures by 7–25% in 3 years (McClung, 1999). In fact, recent evidence showing that the addition of supplemental calcium to alendronate treatment had no effect resulted in a statistically significant, additional reduction in NT_x – a commonly used bone resorption marker (Curr Med Res Opin, 2007). However, as expected, we find that speakers in international symposia representing different drug companies that produce expensive anti-osteoporosis agents seldom highlight the importance of calcium and vitamin D.

In both prevention and treatment of osteoporosis, adequate dietary calcium and vitamin D is necessary to maintain the skeleton, other expensive anti-osteoporosis drug therapies assumes a calcium- and vitamin D-replete patient (NIH, 2000). In a just published important meta-analysis in Lancet, the author after analyzing 29 randomized trials, concluded that current evidence supports the use of calcium, or calcium in combination with vitamin D in the preventive treatment of osteoporosis in people aged 50 or over. For best therapeutic effect, the recommended minimum dose is 1200 mg of calcium, and 800 I.U (instead of the current 400 I.U) of vitamin D (Eslick GD et al., Lancet 2007)

The importance of ensuring a calcium- and vitamin D-replete patient is that calcium and vitamin D intake modulate age-related increases in the PTH levels of bone resorption and occult PTH increases contribute to the pathogenesis of osteoporosis and lessen the effects of anti-osteoporosis medications, and cannot be over-emphasized.

Present Case Scenario

Recall that the normal level of vitamin D in healthy individuals should reach > 30 ng/ml, together with calcium 1,200–1,500 mg per day. $CaCo_3$ is least expensive; Ca citrate is given for those patients on acid inhibitors.

In this case, Francis was taken off all her calcium and vitamin D by the young doctor, she seldom goes out of her home for she is afraid of falling, and seldom has any sun exposure. In effect, there is little difference from the situation of someone living in nursing home, and it is not surprising the vitamin D level was nearly undetectable. The literature has it that vitamin D levels tend to be even lower during winter in many cold countries because of lack of sunshine, and people seldom go out of their homes. In this case, Francis fractured her hip in winter. Finally, you gave Francis a loading dose of vitamin D, together with calcium supplementation in addition to treating her hip fracture. The options available in patients with a break-through fragility fracture, despite being on bisphosphonate therapy will be discussed separately in another case scenario.

Learning Point

- Vitamin D plays an important role in the regulation of calcium levels and bone mineralisation. Its deficiency causes osteomalacia or rickets, while its insufficiency can exacerbate osteoporosis.

- Other important roles include improving gait balance strength, particularly in the elderly, and its effect on the immune system. In addition, the Framingham Study revealed that low intake and low serum level of vitamin D are in fact associated with increased risk of OA progression.

- In countries with a high fracture incidence, a minimum of 400–500 mg of calcium intake is required to prevent osteoporosis. When consumption of dairy products is limited, other sources of calcium include fish with edible bones, tortillas processed with lime, green vegetables high in calcium (e.g., broccoli, kale), legumes and by-products of legumes (e.g., tofu).

- The prevalence of vitamin D deficiency is high, and the situation is especially significant in nursing homes and those community-dwelling elders who are afraid to go outdoors owing to previous falls. Adequate calcium intake from the diet or as a supplement is important for vitamin D to work.

- It is sad that many an orthopedic surgeon either think that both calcium and vitamin D are nothing more than supplements, and an occasional one may even think these are useless. It is time our younger generation of orthopedic surgeons learnt to appreciate more the great importance of calcium and vitamin D, and not just the increasing number of "anti-osteoporosis medications" popularised by the pharmaceutical companies who are in the habit of providing hearty luncheon and dinner receptions to sell their line of products.

- Young surgeons should be reminded of the WHO's Consultation on Mineral Requirements in Human Nutrition report, which made it very clear that in countries with high fracture incidence, increases in dietary vitamin D and calcium in the older populations can decrease fracture risk. Therefore, an adequate vitamin D status should be ensured. If vitamin D is obtained predominantly from dietary sources, for example, when sunshine exposure is limited, an intake of 5–10 g per day is recommended.

- As for associated life-style modifications, the above authority recommends an increase in physical activity; a reduction in sodium intake (excess Na may have a diuretic effect causing more calcium loss in the urine); increased consumption of fruits and vegetables; maintaining a healthy body weight/BMI; avoiding smoking; and limiting alcohol intake. Convincing evidence also indicates that lifetime weight-bearing aerobic physical activity, in particular activity that maintains or increases muscle strength is encouraged.

References

1. World Health Organization. Vitamin and mineral requirements in human nutrition. Report of the Joint FAO/WHO Expert Consultation. Geneva, World Health Organization

2. Utiger RD (1998) The need for more vitamin D. N Engl J Med, 19; 338(12):828–9

3. Bonnick S, Broy S, et al. (2007) Treatment with alendronate plus calcium, alendronate alone, or calcium alone for postmenopausal low bone mineral density. Curr Med Res Opin, 23(6): 1341–9

4. Eslick GD, Tang BM et al (2007) Use of calcium in combination with vitamin D to prevent fractures and bone loss in people aged 50 or older: a meta-analysis. Lancet, 370(9588): 657–66

A Professor Suffering from OA Knee Pain

History and Examination

You were approached one day by your old Australian friend Mr Jones, a 65-year-old retired university associate professor of anatomy and a highly educated and respected teacher at the local university. He told you that after his retirement, he left USA to return to Perth where he owns a big house with a lovely garden. However, he noticed increasing right knee pain made worse by walking stairs, especially downstairs. The local clinic doctor arranged radiographs of his knees, told him he has bilateral knee osteoarthritis more on the right, affecting the right knee medial compartment mainly and by nature is an idiopathic disease. The clinic doctor prescribed a few weeks of painkillers, and a course of physiotherapy, which only partially relieved the knee symptoms. Mr Jones did not have any history of trauma to his knees all these years, and the pain had been getting worse over the past 3 months, and he flew back to US to seek your treatment. Your friend Mr Jones has meanwhile exhausted all the information he could get from the internet concerning his osteoarthritis and he is positive that more can be done about his knees than what he has received so far. Explain how you would manage the right knee pain of Mr Jones who has very high expectations from a rehabilitation specialist like yourself, and how you would brief him about the latest advances in this disease process, which is so common-place. Also, Mr Jones commented that he has doubts about comments made by the clinic doctor that his OA is due to aging; his friend Mr Harrington is nearly 90 years of age, but does not have any knee problems at all. How will you proceed from here?

Discussion

Introduction

Firstly, Mr Jones must be aware that there are fundamental differences between age-related changes of the joint as opposed to osteoarthritis. Old age is not always automatically associated with joint osteoarthritis, although it is regarded as a predisposing factor by many experts. What is more, some patients have joint arthritis, which may be remarkable on radiographs, but can in fact be entirely free of symptoms. In addition, as far as the OA knee is concerned, recent radiological studies demonstrated important ethnic differences in the common patterns of OA changes in the knee between patients in the People's Republic of China, and the Caucasian population in Australia (ORS Proceedings 2007), this point was alluded to earlier in this book.

The histological changes of OA are different from those of normal chronic use of the joint, as this professor of anatomy is fully aware.

In addition, many of us are aware that many human diseases are the result of a complex interaction between genetics and environment. Environmental factors are easy to perceive. In a large series of knee arthroscopy reported by Shelbourne and others in the past, the incidence of chondral lesions, many of which are asymptomatic, can be as high as 40–50% and extensive or multiple sizable chondral lesions, particularly if left untreated, can predispose to a more generalized osteoarthritic process. Thus, we will first discuss the normal control of chondrocyte and matrix signaling, followed by current models of injury leading to osteoarthritis, and finally talk about the rapid advances in the understanding of genetic factors.

Basic Concepts of Chondrocyte/Matrix Functionality/Signaling

Much of the new knowledge of this aspect has come about in recent years after investigating cartilage on the nano-scale via the use of atomic force microscopy and piezo-electric instruments, and is summarized in point form here for simplicity:

- Concept 1: Articular chondrocytes respond to both chemical and mechanical signaling, depending on their zone of origin (the zones have been described in the companion texts by the author), and with respect to the distance from the surface of the cartilage.

- Concept 2: It was through the use of advanced instruments like atomic force microscopy that we have begun to understand the biological functionality of this avascular, aneural (without nerves), tissue known as cartilage.

- Concept 3: The mechanical stimuli mentioned above include the deformation of cell and matrix, fluid flow, hydrostatic pressure, alteration of intra- or peri-cellular pH, electrical streaming potential, and so forth. Mechanical signals can influence chondrocyte matrix metabolism via signaling, transcription, translation, as well as their effect on post-translation modification.

- Concept 4: Static compression tends to inhibit the synthesis of collagen, aggrecan, and small proteoglycan. However, dynamic compression stimulates extracellular matrix molecules; and dynamic shear stimulates the biosynthesis of collagen.

- Concept 5: Thus, the exact joint-loading environment has a large influence on chondrocyte gene expression. Nowadays, we hear many different research groups trying to use different 3D scaffolding plus cell seeding (including the use of, say, mesenchymal stem cells) to regenerate a damaged cartilage surface, the majority claiming a good result. However, the crux of the matter boils down to:
  - Whether this kind of signaling function of the new tissue is re-established with the nearby native tissue (to prevent future arthrosis)
  - Investigating on the nano scale via the use of atomic force or piezo-electric instruments and microscopy to see the practical functionality of the new tissue, and not just the "appearance" on a second-look arthroscopy.

- Concept 6: While traumatic joint injuries are known to increase the risk of osteoarthritis, the mechanism is not known. What we do know is that injurious compression can significantly up-regulate gene expression of aggrecanese-2 (ADAMTS-5) and stromelysin (MMP-3) mRNA, as well as protein levels of catabolic factors. Mechanical injury induces damage to the tissue matrix directly or mediated by chondrocytes via expression of matrix-degrading enzymes and reduction of biosynthetic activity. The expression of several matrix-degrading enzymes like ADAM-TS5 and matrix-metalloproteinases (MMP-1, MMP-2, MMP-3, MMP-9, MMP-13) is also increased after injury and may in part be regulated by an autocrine vascular endothelial growth factor (VEGF)-dependent signaling pathway. Apoptosis seems to be mediated by caspase activity and reactive oxygen species. For that reason, activation of antioxidative defense mechanisms as well as the inhibition of angiogenetic factors and MMPs may be key regulators in the mechanically induced destruction of cartilage and could be suggested as potential therapeutic interventions of the future.

■ Concept 7: The presence of catabolic cytokines after joint injury may significantly alter cell response to even normal physiological levels of loading. Injured cartilaginous tissue may not respond to the normal stimulatory effects of moderate dynamic compression.

Stages of Formation of the Osteoarthritic Process

■ Stage 1: High impact loading or other causes disrupt the matrix macromolecular structure – resulting in more water and less proteoglycan aggregate.

■ Stage 2: Chondrocytes detect the tissue damage and release mediators that stimulate a cellular response – both anabolic and catabolic activities increased together with increased cellularity (which might explain why in some cases the process may improve/abort/revert). The histology involves "clones of proliferating cells surrounded by newly synthesized matrix molecules, which is a typical hallmark".

■ Stage 3: Progression of cartilage loss and abated anabolic response. There are additional two areas of interest here:
  • Changes in the subchondral area – increased density, cyst formation, cyst cavities with myxoid/fibrous/cartilage tissues together with the appearance of regenerating cartilage within and on the subchondral bone surface. At the end stage, there is thick dense bone-on-bone articulation.
  • Formation of osteophytes – around the periphery of joints – marginal at the "cartilage-bone interface" and along the insertions of the joint capsule (capsular osteophytes). Most marginal osteo-

phytes have a cartilaginous surface that resembles normal articular cartilage, and looks like an extension of the joint surface.

Genetic Factor

As far as the genetic factor is concerned, the situation is more complex. In the past 10 years, a large number of twin-pair, sibling-risk and segregation studies have been conducted on osteoarthritis, and these have revealed a major genetic component that is transmitted in a non-mendelian manner. OA therefore fits best into the complex, multifactorial class of common diseases. With a genetic component established, genome-wide linkage scans were performed, and these finally uncovered several genomic intervals likely to harbor OA susceptibility. In the past few years these intervals have started to yield genes containing OA-associated variants. The genes that have so far been implicated in OA susceptibility include the interleukin 1 gene (IL1) cluster at chromosome 2q11.2-q13, the matrilin 3 gene (MATN3) at 2p24.1, the IL-4 receptor alpha-chain gene (IL4R) at 16p12.1, the secreted frizzled-related protein 3 gene (FRZB) at 2q32.1, the metalloproteinase gene ADAM12 at 10q26.2 and, most recently, the asporin gene (ASPN) at 9q22.31.

The evidence of involvement of these genes in OA is more compelling for some than for others, with the IL1 and ASPN associations being the most convincing to date, according to research from Nuffield Oxford, Japan and elsewhere. The gene products of IL1, IL4R, FRZB and ASPN regulate cartilage chondrocyte differentiation and survival, and their effects on the chondrocyte may potentially be amenable to therapeutic intervention in the future (Loughlin, J Expert Rev Mol Med, 2005).

Asporin is an extracellular matrix component expressed abundantly in the articular cartilage of OA patients. A significant association between a polymorphism in the aspartic acid (D) repeat of the asporin gene (ASPN) and knee OA was found; the D14 allele of ASPN is over-represented relative to the common D13 allele, and its frequency increases with disease severity. The D14 allele is also over-represented in patients with hip OA. The association of asporin is replicated in the European population by meta-analysis. Asporin suppresses transforming growth factor-beta (TGF-β)-mediated expression of aggrecan and type II collagen genes and reduced proteoglycan accumulation in an in vitro model of chondrogenesis. Asporin co-localized to and bound to TGF-β, and inhibited TGF-β-Smad signal. Clarification of the molecular pathway of OA relating to asporin and TGF-β would lead to order-made medicine and novel therapeutic strategies for OA (Ikegawa, Clin Calcium, 2006).

It was further reported that an aspartic acid (D)-repeat polymorphism in the gene encoding asporin (ASPN) was associated with OA of knee and hip joints in Japanese; in the three independent studies performed, the D14 allele of the ASPN polymorphism was over-represented, and the D13 allele was under-represented. Subsequently, four replication studies, three in European and one in Chinese populations, have been reported.

In hip OA, significant heterogeneity was identified and there was no positive association for any allele in any comparison. The present results suggest that the association of the ASPN D14 allele and knee OA has global relevance, but that its effect has ethnic differences (Nakamura et al., Hum Mol Genet, 2007).

Management of Mr Jones

You found on careful examination that Mr Jones has mild to moderate right knee genu varum with pain mainly over the medial side of the right knee; his quadriceps power was reasonable, and there was no effusion. There was mild restriction of ROM, and the radiographs revealed a mainly antero-medial pattern of OA changes. Mr Jones expressed that he does not want any surgery.

After patient education, you referred Mr Jones for a course of pain-relieving physiotherapy, followed by joint unloading knee braces (Fig. 20) to unload the mainly arthritic right medial knee compartment, as there is recent literature in support of unloading knee braces in predominant uni-compartmental knee arthritis (J Knee Surg, 2002). Mr Jones then received a course of hydrotherapy and under-water walking training after pain subsided, which was guided by a trained therapist. Functional rehabilitation then followed and catered for maneuvers that he found difficult to handle in daily living such as sitting to standing, or squatting,

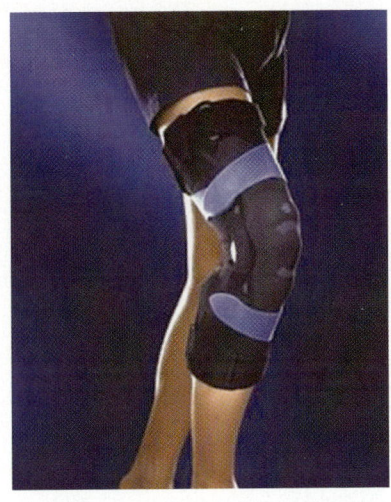

Fig. 20 Unloading knee braces such as the one illustrated may help partly relieve the joint loading on the medial knee compartment (courtesy of Donjoy)

etc., with the help of both physiotherapist and occupational therapist. You also stressed the importance of a healthy life-style, weight control, chronic life-long weight-bearing exercises, staying active and considering Tai Chi exercises. Incidentally, Tai Chi has just been shown in gait laboratory studies in the USA to improve gait, stability in one-legged stance, and stability in negotiating over obstacles (Gait Posture, 2007). You reminded Mr Jones to avoid smoking and alcohol, and to ensure adequate calcium and vitamin D to maintain bone health; the latter may also help prevent OA progression according to recent research, as reported in ORS Proceedings, 2007.

Learning Point

- Osteoarthritis is not and should *not* be regarded as the end result of aging changes in the synovial joint of the knee, although old age may be regarded as a predisposing factor.

- In other words, aging is likely to be one of the necessary, but not sufficient conditions for the process of osteoarthritis to occur. Other modulating factors include genetic factors of which the asporin and IL1 genes are important and mechanical factors like joint trauma (macro- or repeated micro-trauma), and alteration of the mechanical axis may act as precipitating or perpetuating factors.

- Unlike rheumatoid arthritis, where there are lots of disease-modifying drugs, including new agents like remicade, there is as yet no pharmacological agent that can reliably alter the natural history of osteoarthritis once generalised osteoarthritis sets in. The role of glucosamine and hyaluronan have been discussed separately in this book.

- For knees with a mild degree of varus and mainly medial compartment knee pain when walking or not with an adduction moment, and the arthrosis is not so far advanced that it warrants immediate surgery or if surgery is refused by patient, the author advises the use of corrective joint unloading knee braces to lessen the force transmission across the medial compartment, besides exercises guided by physiotherapists, weight loss, life-style modification, and hydrotherapy.

- There is increasing support for the use of Tai Chi exercise in improving gait in the elderly, including the just reported gait laboratory objective studies. However, one should caution our patients with knee OA not to practise the one-legged Tai Chi manoeuvres during painful flare-ups of the knee joint.

References

1. Ikegawa S (2006) Asporin, a susceptibility gene for osteoarthritis. Clin Calcium Sep, 16(9):1548–52
2. Nakamura T, Shi D, et al. (2007) Meta-analysis of association between the ASPN D-repeat and osteoarthritis. Hum Mol Genet, 16:1676–81

3. Loughlin J (2005) The genetic epidemiology of human primary osteoarthritis: Current status. Expert Rev Mol Med, 24; 7(9):1–12

4. Paulos LE, Finger S (2002) Clinical and biomechanical evaluation of the unloading knee brace. J Knee Surg, 15(3):155–8

5. Einhorn T (2006) Orthopaedic basic science. American Academy of Orthopaedic Surgeons Press

6. Ramachandran AK, Rosengren KS, et al. (2007) Effect of Tai Chi on gait and obstacle crossing behaviors in middle-aged adults. Gait Posture, 26(2):248–255

History and Examination

Mrs Andrews is a 39-year-old housewife living in Florida. She lives with her husband and two children. Three years ago, she started to notice pins and needles in her right hand. The numbness was poorly localized. She was seen and followed up by her family doctor, who provided symptomatic treatment in terms of vitamins and some blood checks and reassurance. Only when Mrs Andrews' symptoms got worse was she referred to a local orthopod 1 year ago. She was variously treated by night-time splintage, vitamins, and radiograph examination of the cervical spine and thoracic outlets. As the patience of Mrs Andrews was wearing thin after not being given a definitive diagnosis, she asked for a second opinion and went to your clinic instead. The partner of your private practice examined Mrs Andrews on the first clinic visit and he wrote down the following in the case notes: Mrs Andrews did not have any gross muscle wasting, the Adson's and Spurling's tests were both negative. The upper and lower limb jerks were normal. There was no numbness in the dermatomal or glove and stocking distribution. Signs of cervical myelopathy were absent. Tinel's sign was positive on the right side, but Phalen's sign was negative. Mrs Andrews asked your partner what the diagnosis was exactly. Your colleague answered by saying she probably has carpal tunnel syndrome, especially since recent radiographs of the cervical spine and thoracic outlets were unremarkable. To play safe, he considered MRI of the cervical spine for further investigation. As for the suspected carpal tunnel syndrome, he considered booking elective nerve conduction testing for Mrs Andrews and surgery will be considered if conservative treatment fails.

During the next clinic visit, you saw Mrs Andrews, who, as expected, did not improve with "conservative management" and was getting even more impatient. You found the recently described "on-profile" sign of carpal tunnel syndrome to be positive on bedside examination. Mrs Andrews stood up out of the chair exclaiming how it was possible that she herself did not notice the wasting of her own right hand in the past. You subsequently arranged a fast-track appointment for nerve conduction testing the following week and scheduled Mrs Andrews for surgery 2 weeks later. Postoperatively, her numbness was completely relieved, but she was still wondering why it took as long as 3 years for a diagnosis to be made and proper treatment initiated.

Discussion

It should be stressed that while late and severe muscle wasting is easy to see on inspection of the patient's hands in an AP direction as traditionally taught in old textbooks, these cases represent late cases where the thenar muscles are chronically denervated and too late for salvage. It is the identification of *early* thenar muscle wasting therefore that is important. But the author noticed over the years that many a clinician misses the early muscle wasting that can be seen by properly re-positioning both hands of the patient in about 50–70° pronation during examination instead of the AP direction (Fig. 21) as taught in old traditional textbooks. The author coined this test the "On Profile" test for carpal tunnel syndrome.

The loss of the smooth contour of the thenar eminence of the hand is made very obvious when both hands are thus re-positioned (Fig. 22).

Very frequently, when the author showed this sign to an affected patient, he/she immediately jumped up from the chair asking how it was possible that the wasting had gone unnoticed for the past few years, and queried why the clinicians treating her never showed the subtle muscle wasting to the patient. The other good point about showing this physical sign to the patient is that it becomes much easier to convince the patient that operative intervention is needed, as muscle wasting is present.

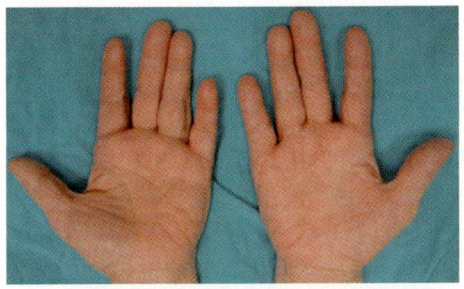

Fig. 21 Viewed in the traditionally taught antero-posterior direction, the thenar eminence muscles appear unremarkable

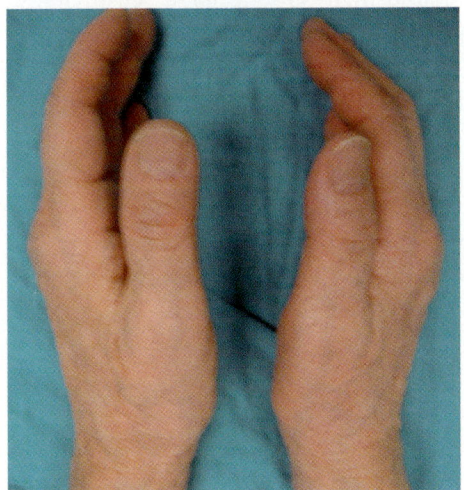

Fig. 22 Viewed in 50° pronation of both forearms immediately brings out subtle wasting usually of the abductor pollicis brevis muscle, constituting a positive "on-profile" sign

A recent Canadian study showed a large amount of permanent pain and suffering, significant loss of work productivity, and considerable financial cost as a result of work-related CTS in an article entitled: "Carpal tunnel syndrome: cross-sectional and outcome study in Ontario workers" (Manktelow et al., J Hand Surg [Am], 2004), and stresses the importance of *early* detection and intervention of cases that require surgery.

Detection of early muscle wasting with the help of the new physical sign as described here aids decision-making to persuade the patient to go for surgery instead of procrastination.

Learning Point

- The newly described "On Profile" sign in CTS is particularly useful for front-line workers like junior residents as well as primary care physicians. Detection of a positive sign in the former case needs consultation with a senior colleague with a view to surgery to prevent further muscle atrophy, while detection of the same in the case of primary care physicians warrants referral to an orthopaedic unit for surgery without hesitation. The author found high (around 90%) sensitivity and specificity of this test for the diagnosis of moderate CTS that warrants surgery (paper submitted for publication).

- Recent large-scale studies of CTS in Canada showed a large amount of permanent pain and suffering, significant loss of work productivity, and considerable financial cost as a result of work-related CTS. These workers, who are frequently the breadwinner of the family should be relieved of the suffering *early* to prevent work loss and further muscle wasting.

References

1. Ip D (2007) Orthopedic rehabilitation, assessment, and enablement, Springer, Heidelberg
2. Manktelow RT, Binhammer P, et al. (2004) Carpal tunnel syndrome: cross-sectional and outcome study in Ontario workers. J Hand Surg (Am), 29(2):307–17

History and Examination

William is a 36-year-old heavy manual laborer working on car parts assembly line, and a person of strong muscle build. Nearly 2 years ago, owing to machinery malfunction, William was hit on the back by one of the car parts. William required 3 weeks of hospitalization before he was sufficiently well to ambulate again, after 3 weeks of intense physiotherapy. Radiograph of the lumbar spine did not reveal any fractures, and MRI of the lumbar spine was negative. At 6 months post-injury, your colleague working in another hospital referred him to have medical board assessment. However, William refused – thinking that he had not attained the state of maximal medical improvement, although William expressed the strong wish to return to his previous workplace. Your colleague then referred William for a course of work hardening and work rehabilitation. This was followed by a short work trial in which William tried to return to his workplace for a few hours each day to see whether he could cope. This did not work out and back pain and poor endurance was thought to be the cause of failure to return to work. Your colleague then referred him for a further course of work hardening using Baltimore Therapeutic Equipment, but the effect was fair and this situation lingered on for yet another half a year. Finally, the employer asked a private occupational therapist to perform the now very popular "functional capacity evaluation" on William. The FCE report was in favor of William being able to return to work in the capacity of moderately heavy to heavy demand jobs. Two months later, after finishing all the work hardening together with an extra course of hydrotherapy, William returned to his workplace and was given a moderate demand job. However, 3 weeks later, William quickly had a relapse of his back pain and was on sick leave again. Then followed several months of mainly back pain followed by a brief return to work and pain again. Frustrated by the lack of progress, your colleague referred William to be assessed by a rehabilitation specialist like you. Describe how you would tackle this case scenario of chronic back pain with much disability, and comment whether you are surprised to find in this case that FCE failed to accurately predict William's ability to return to work.

Discussion

Back pain is a very common cause of failure to return to work in injury on duty claims. There is an increasing number of employers, insurance companies, disability management case managers, and even attorneys who rely on the now popular "functional capacity evaluation" (FCE), claiming it may serve as an objective test for predicting whether the patient will be able to cope.

Before we talk about FCE and its pitfalls, let us first reveal the case at hand. One should first note from the teachings of the companion textbook by the same author that back pain should be actively dealt with and followed up in the acute and subacute stage, since if chronicity sets in, as in this case, it is much more difficult to treat.

In the present case scenario, there are certain insufficiencies in management by your colleague before the patient gets referred to you. This includes:

- No work-place visit or job analysis
- No multi-disciplinary team was arranged to tackle this chronic pain patient with constant feedback and conferencing
- Lack of adequate work-up of possible psychological and social factors that may contribute to the perpetuation of the pain

In the companion textbook by the same author, recall that there is a proposed renewed definition of pain as follows: "Pain refers to an unpleasant sensory and emotional experience (that may be associated with actual or feeling of potential tissue damage) and which is characterized frequently by special pain behavior, the latter being determined by personal, physical and social context of the individual in question". Examples of personal factors, such as the patient's own beliefs are affected by his mind and past learned experiences, while examples of social factors include the behavior and beliefs of his relatives and family.

Examples of the Importance of Pain Behavior in Chronic Pain
Evidence from the fear avoidance model of chronic pain (i.e. disability is largely determined by the erroneous belief that an increase in activity level is potentially harmful): recent research has found a relationship between self-reported disability and fear avoidance beliefs, by demonstrating the relationship of fear of work to actual work-related behavior (Vowles and Gross, Pain, 2003). In a recent paper entitled: "Assessment of chronic pain behavior: reliability of the method and its relationship with perceived disability, physical impairment and function", it was found that there was a strong correlation between pain behavior (studied as a video-based assessment) and subjective pain report and disability. The author further concluded that pain and pain behavior were the two most important determinants of self-reported disability (Koho et al., J Rehabil Med, 2001).

Comprehensive Assessment of Pain Behavior in this Patient
In the present case scenario, we used the following for assessment:
- Self-report of disability and pain intensity were assessed using the Oswestry disability questionnaire (better than the Roland Morris for chronic severe disability)
- The pain visual analogue scale (VAS)
- Depression and somatic perception were assessed using the modified somatic perception questionnaire
- The Tampa scale for kinesiophobia was used to evaluate fear of movement and (re)injury
- Video-based assessment with playback

Result of Assessment of this Clinical Case

In this case, William's problems turn out to be not fear avoidance, but to kinesiophobia, which is not an uncommon condition among patients with musculoskeletal pain conditions (Lundberg et al., J Rehabil Med, 2006).

Fear of movement and re-injury (kinesiophobia) has been postulated to play an important role in the performance in an FCE. In a recent study in the literature performed to analyze the relationship between kinesiophobia and performance in an FCE setting, kinesiophobia and FCE performance of 54 male and 10 female patients suffering chronic low back pain in a recent study from the Netherlands. The researchers commented that: "…the results indicate that the patients were substantially kinesiophobic, yet they were able to lift a mean of 29.5 kg and were physically able to perform moderate to heavy work." (Reneman et al., J Occup Rehabil, 2003).

Reliability of FCE Results in Predicting Ability to RTW in Chronic LBP

- Better performance on evaluation was only weakly associated with faster recovery in workers with chronic LBP as shown recently by Gross and Batt (Spine, 2004).
- Contrary to functional capacity evaluation theory, better functional capacity evaluation performance – as indicated by a lower number of failed tasks – was in fact associated not infrequently with higher risk of recurrence. The validity of FCE in accurately predicting and in identifying workers deemed "safe" to return to work is suspect (Gross and Batt, Spine, 2004).

Management

- Philips reported in Behav Res Ther (1991) the positive effect of behavioral counseling within a problem-solving content to encourage exercise, socialization, and return to work. These results were better than psychotherapy alone in terms of pain resolution and return to daily activities.
- In the present case scenario, besides behavioral counseling, William recovered after a full course of psychotherapy by the psychiatrist in the multi-disciplinary team.

Learning Point

■ As orthopedic surgeons, we do come across the need to write up medical reports as requested by employers or insurance companies for workers injured on duty suffering from chronic LBP. Often, they come with an FCE report in hand. This case illustrates that use of FCE as a method of predicting ability to return to work in laborers has limitations, at least as shown here that kinesiophobic individuals may spuriously be commented upon in the FCE report to be able to perform moderate to heavy work.

■ Diagnosis of kinesiophobia is not always straightforward. In this case, diagnosis was made after the Tampa scale for kinesiophobia for evaluation of fear of movement and (re)injury, as well as video-based assessment with playback.

■ A biopsychosocial approach is usually successful in managing patients with kinesiophobia.

References

1. Koho P, Aho S, et al. (2001) Assessment of chronic pain behaviour: reliability of the method and its relationship with perceived disability, physical impairment and function. J Rehabil Med, 33(3):128–132

2. Vowles KE, Gross RT (2003) Work-related beliefs about injury and physical capacity for work in individuals with chronic pain. Pain, 101(3):291–298

3. Gross DP, Batt MC (2004) The prognostic value of functional capacity evaluation in patients with chronic low back pain. II. Sustained recovery. Spine 29(8):920–924

4. Lundberg M, Larsson M, et al. (2006) Kinesiophobia among patients with musculoskeletal pain in primary healthcare. J Rehabil Med, 38(1):37–43

Breakthrough Fracture While on Bisphosphonates

History and Examination

Veronica is a well-bred university lecturer in her late sixties who went from sunny San Diego where she used to work to join her grandmother who lives in New York after retirement. Veronica has all along led a healthy lifestyle, and strives to stay in shape by jogging. She is a non-smoker and non-drinker, and has good medical health except a history of partial thyroidectomy for a benign thyroid growth on thyroxine replacement, and one episode of deep vein thrombosis after a long flight to the Philippines on holiday. She suffered from a fractured L2 vertebra (Grade 2 on Genant's scale) during winter 2 years ago after having a fall amid a snow blizzard that hit the New York and Boston district. A local New York hospital tackled her wedge collapse of L2 with attempted cement vertebroplasty electively, but this was aborted due to leakage of cement, and she was given a 6-week course of intensive physiotherapy after which she made a prompt recovery. A DXA scan showed a T-score of –2.5 and she was given bisphosphonates by an attending physiatrist together with some calcium and vitamin D tablets. Her ambulatory status quickly improved and she could resume most of the daily activities 3 months after discharge. Her thyroid function tests came back as entirely normal.

Veronica had good compliance with her medication, which consisted of weekly alendronate initially, then changed to monthly ibandronate (Bonviva). However, Veronica suffered a fractured right neck of the femur 6 weeks ago after losing balance on the supermarket's wet floor, despite 2 years of anti-osteoporosis treatment. After fixation of Veronica's fracture with cemented bipolar hemiarthroplasty, Veronica requested that you analyzed her osteoporosis treatment in detail and whether bisphosphonates really work for her.

Discussion

There are three issues as regards bisphosphonates therapy as an anti-osteoporosis agent. First, Veronica should note that taking bisphosphonates like alendronate or risedronate, even in the presence of adequate calcium and vitamin D intake, although it may decrease the chance of both vertebral and non-vertebral fractures, it does not eliminate the possibility of each and every fragility fracture occurring. Second, we understand that she had been shifted to receive the newer, more potent, long-acting ibandronate (Bonviva) and had been doing so for some time. There is some support in the literature for this new ibandronate in preventing vertebral fractures, and some non-vertebral ones, but the efficacy of Bonviva in preventing hip fractures (like the one Veronica suffers in this episode) is not yet proven beyond doubt. Third, not each and every patient has the expected positive increase in bone mass after bisphosphonates treatment, even in the presence of a calcium-/vitamin D-replete scenario and assuming good drug compliance. That is why sometimes we do a DXA 1 year after the start of bisphosphonates.

Tackling "Break-through" Fractures Despite Being on Bisphosphonates: Options

- Option 1: do nothing, observe. Treat the hip fracture, continue the bisphosphonate treatment. The current recommendation for bisphosphonates therapy is to continue for more than 5 years and up to 10 years. There are no data after the 10-year mark, i.e., whether too prolonged therapy will increase bone brittleness from over-suppression of bone re-modeling is unsure even among experts at this stage since there are no data beyond the 10-year mark.
- Option 2: Doing a biochemical screen in these cases is advisable and is the usual practice of the author when he encounters breakthrough fractures while on bisphosphonates. This biochemical work-up includes: assay of Ca PO4, 1,25-di(OH) vitamin D, 24 h urinary calcium, bone formation markers like ALP, and bone resorption markers like NTX (N-telopeptide).

- Option 3: Consideration should also be given to switching to other treatment choices like strontium, or pulsatile PTH therapy, which are to be discussed in the following sections.

Treatment Options if Switching of Therapy Decided Upon

- SERM – not advisable here since Veronica has a history of deep vein thrombosis
- Strontium renelate
- Pulsatile Forteo (teriparatide)

Strontium

Despite the fact that an occasional expert in osteoporosis commented that the mechanism of action of strontium ranelate is largely unknown, studies from France have suggested that strontium has the *dual* action of simultaneously increasing bone formation and decreasing bone re-sorption (Marie, Curr Opin Rheumatol, 2006). This comes about via a simultaneous increase in the replication of pre-osteoblasts, resulting in an increase in osteoblasts, as well as a decrease in the differentiation of pre-osteoclasts into osteoclasts and a decrease in the bone resorption action of osteoclasts. Despite the aforementioned, many researchers feel that in humans as opposed to animal models, the bone formation stimulation effect may actually be less than in animals.

Role in non-vertebral fracture reduction: In a recent multi-center TROPOS (treatment of peripheral osteoporosis study) trial involving most European countries and some Scandinavian countries, as far as non-vertebral fractures are concerned; the authors found that the relative risk of experiencing a hip fracture in the ITT (intention-to-treat) population was reduced by 15% but that this figure did not reach statistical significance, as this study was not designed nor powered for this parameter. However, it was found in a *post-hoc* analysis that in the high-risk fracture subgroup, i.e., of older ladies > 74 years with femoral neck BMD T-score ≤ -3.0; treatment was associated with a 36% reduction in risk of hip fracture (Reginster et al., J Clin Endocrinol Metab, 2005).

Regarding its role in vertebral fracture reduction, risk reduction was demonstrated in both the TROPOS trial mentioned above as well as an earlier SOTI study (spinal osteoporosis therapeutic intervention). The latter involved 1,649 post-menopausal ladies, and a dose of strontium ranelate at 2 g per day orally reduced the relative risk of new vertebral fracture by 49% at 1 year and 41% over 3 years (Meunier et al., N Engl J Med, 2004).

In a Cochrane Review for strontium ranelate (2006), the authors commented that there is evidence to support the efficacy of strontium ranelate for the reduction of fractures (vertebral and to a lesser extent non-vertebral) in postmenopausal osteoporotic women. Diarrhea may occur, however, and adverse events leading to study withdrawal were not significantly increased with taking 2 g of strontium ranelate daily. Potential vascular and neurological side effects need to be further explored in future studies.

Pulsatile Forteo or Teriparatide Treatment

Endocrinologists previously found that continuous high-dose PTH infusion causes a catabolic effect on bones; while a low-dose once daily administration will have anabolic effects instead.

This anabolic effect of a PTH once-daily dose comes about by means of stimulation of the bone-lining cells, decreased RANKL, increased OPG, decreased osteoblast apoptosis, and possibly also stimulates BMP, IGF, cbfa1 and Wnt signaling. The overall effect results in enhanced osteoblast function and population, thus with a positive effect on bone formation. This anabolic action *outweighs* the stimulation of osteoclasts, which is believed to be mediated via interleukin-6 gene expression in a previous animal experiment in rats (Chiba et al., J Vet Med Sci, 2002).

The clinical effect of decreased bone resorption markers (e.g., NTx) and increased formation markers (e.g., PINP or amino-terminal propeptide of type 1 pro-collagen) was achieved by teriparatide therapy, but *not* alendronate, as demonstrated in the FACT study (Fig. 23) (McClung et al., Arch Intern Med, 2005).

In fact, studies showed that teriparatide injection once daily also improves bone micro-architecture (Jiang et al., J Bone Min Res, 2003) in the form of better trabecular volume, cortical thickness, and better connectivity on checking serial transiliac crest bone biopsies, plus an

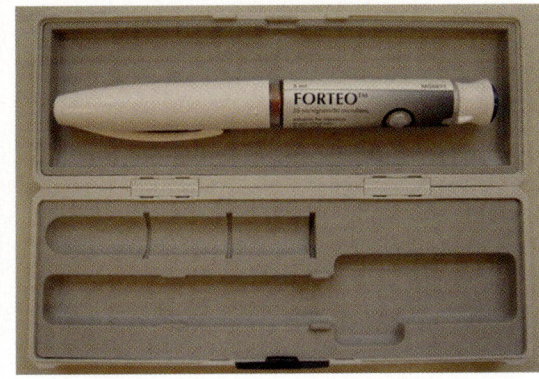

Fig. 23 The drug teriparatide, commercially marketed as "Forteo"

improved mineralization pattern (Misof et al., J Clin Endocrinol Metab, 2003).

However, potential patients should be cautioned that Forteo *cannot* be given with bisphosphonates (as they act in opposite actions) and patients should be cautioned that osteosarcoma was reported in animals, although no human cases were found and FDA has approved its use. Monitoring of serum Ca is needed, however.

In addition, while bisphosphonates need to be given for at least 5–10 years according to the finding of the FLEX study, Forteo needs to be given for only 18 months. Forteo is particularly indicated in severe osteoporosis, but the treatment cost is high.

SERM

SERM stands for "selective estrogen receptor modulators". As the name implies, they are not compounds like the pure anti-estrogens (e.g., ICI 182, 780), which antagonize the effect of estrogens in all tissues including bone, uterus, breast, and cardiovascular system.

Different classes of SERMs exhibit *both* agonist as well as antagonist effects on the above tissue, depending on the tissue in question and the hormonal milieu. The estrogen receptor changes its shape when there is binding by SERM, the resultant shape will then determine which gene will be activated, hence the type of proteins produced (Yang et al., Science, 1996).

The only type of SERM licensed to manage osteoporosis are the benzothiophene derivative (e.g., raloxifene), but SERM is probably *not* indicated for our patient since she has a history of deep vein thrombosis and SERM is more useful in preventing vertebral rather than non-vertebral fractures, as was shown in the MORE study.

Serial BMD Measurement Arranged for Veronica

- You subsequently switched Veronica to have strontium renelate therapy. Serial BMD testing was arranged for her. Serial BMD can evaluate individuals for non-response by finding loss of bone density, suggesting the need for re-evaluation of treatment and evaluation of the secondary causes of osteoporosis.
- Follow-up BMD testing in situations other than breakthrough fractures despite bisphosphonates should be done whenever the expected change in BMD equals or exceeds the least significant change (LSC) as suggested by ISCD.

Additional Key Concept

Although management of osteoporosis after fragility fractures is important, as one tackles a progressively aging population (in particular patients after the 8th decade), then fall prevention measures becoming equally or not more important, especially if the index fall event was caused by intrinsic factors, as shown by the author (Ip et al., J Orthop Surg, 2006).

Learning Point

- This case scenario illustrates the not uncommon scenario of fragility fractures occurring despite bisphosphonates treatment. In fact, if we calculate the rise in bone mass, we find the rate of increase after teriparatide (Forteo) treatment is quicker than after bisphosphonates.

- Although one may argue that bisphosphonates treatment only reduces the chance of fragility fractures and does not prevent such fractures altogether, still it will be prudent to recheck the compliance, and also bone markers for bone resorption, which, if they remain elevated, despite, say having started the treatment for 1–2 years, may suggest occult causes like secondary hyperparathyroidism from vitamin D insufficiency, hypercalciuria, occult thyroid disease, etc. The issue of whether those patients who have received these medications for over, say, 5 years, need to be discontinued after a breakthrough fracture lest it affects acute bone healing remains an unanswered question.

- Pulsatile Forteo treatment is now FDA-approved; it is usually given to those with fragility fractures and severe osteoporosis, and the usual duration of treatment is 18 months. Forteo should never be given together with bisphosphonates. This is because they have opposite mechanisms of action (McClung MR, San Martin J et al., 2005).

- Strontium has been found to have dual action, but the frequently observed relatively rapid increase in bone mass is partly due to it being a heavy metal. It is usually given at night, and is a definite alternative for those elderly who cannot tolerate bisphosphonates.

- A once-yearly infusion of the potent bisphosphonate zoledronic acid during a 3-year period was recently found to significantly reduce the risk of vertebral, hip, and other fractures (Black et al., N Eng J Med, 2007). However, there are occasional adverse events, including changes in renal function, and serious atrial fibrillation occurred more frequently in the zoledronic acid group than controls; thus, it should be used with caution.

- There is some support of the clinical efficacy of monthly (as opposed to daily) ibandronate – the drug this patient was put on – from the MOBILE study (Miller et al., J Bone Miner Res, 2005). However, the latest study on ibandronate has not yet confirmed its efficacy in fragility hip fracture prevention beyond an element of doubt.

- Even in the just published WHO guidelines on the selection of osteoporosis medications in postmenopausal women, the emerging problem of breakthrough fragility fractures, despite adequate bisphosphonates therapy in a calcium-/vitamin D-replete patient, was not being highlighted (Gorai, Clin Calcium, 2007). This is of practical importance as we expect more and more patients to be put on bisphosphonates.

References

1. McClung MR, San Martin J, et al. (2005) Opposite bone remodeling effects of teriparatide and alendronate in increasing bone mass. Arch Intern Med, 165(15):1762–8

2. Black DM, et al. (2007) A once-yearly infusion of zoledronic acid during a 3-year period significantly reduced the risk of vertebral, hip, and other fractures. N Eng J Med, 556:1809–22

3. Miller PD, McClung MR, et al. (2005) Monthly oral ibandronate therapy in postmenopausal osteoporosis: 1-year results from the MOBILE study. J Bone Miner Res, 20(8):1315–22

4. Marie PJ (2006) Strontium ranelate: a dual mode of action rebalancing bone turnover in favour of bone formation. Curr Opin Rheumatol, 18: suppl 1:S11–5

5. O'Donnell S, Cranney A, et al. (2006) Strontium ranelate for preventing and treating postmenopausal osteoporosis. Cochrane Database Syst Rev, (4):CD005326

6. Reginster JY, Seeman E, et al. (2005) Strontium ranelate reduces the risk of non-vertebral fractures in postmenopausal woman with osteoporosis: TROPOS study. J Clin Endocrinol Metab, 90(5):2816–2822

7. Meunier PJ, Roux C, et al. (2004) The effects of strontium ranelate on the risk of vertebral fracture in women with postmenopausal osteoporosis. N Engl J Med, 350(5):459–468

8. Chiba S, Neer RM, et al. (2002) Parathyroid hormone induces interleukin-6 gene expression in bone stromal cells in rats. J Vet Med Sci, 64(7):641–4

9. Jiang Y, Zhao JJ, et al. (2003) Recombinant human parathyroid hormone (1–34) [teriparatide] improves both cortical and cancellous bone structure. J Bone Min Res, 18(11):1932–41

10. Misof BM, Roschger P, et al. (2003) Effects of intermittent parathyroid hormone administration on bone mineralization density in iliac crest biopsies from patients with osteoporosis – a paired study before and after treatment. J Clin Endocrinol Metab, 88(3):1150–6

11. Yang NN, Venugopalan M, et al. (1996) Identification of an estrogen response element activated by metabolites of 17 beta-estradiol and raloxifene. Science, 273(5279):1222–5

12. Gorai I (2007) Absolute risk for fracture and WHO guideline: selection of drugs for the prevention of fractures in postmenopausal woman. Clin Calcium 17:7, 1090–6

13. Ip D, Ip FK (2006) Elderly patients with two episodes of fragility hip fractures form a special subgroup. J Orthop Surg, 14(3):245–8

Can Back Pain Be Predicted?

History and Examination

Johnathan is a 29-year-old, well-known jockey earning millions each year riding horses, and whom you have treated for a right foot fracture dislocation in the past, and for which he is most grateful. Johnathan has a close colleague by the name of Anthony who is also a jockey and has been having non-traumatic recurrent back pain, which has defied all standard treatment. Johnathan searched the web and there are multiple articles mentioning back pain is commonplace with high recurrence risks and some 80% having an elusive etiology. Getting very nervous, Johnathan went to your office requesting a body check to see whether there is any problem with his back and asks you to assess how likely his chance of getting back pain is. Furthermore, he saw multiple web sites telling of different muscle strengthening exercises to the back written by different athletic trainers and he wants to know whether he needs to indulge himself on these.

Discussion

You told Johnathan that the Danish spine expert, Fin Biering-Sorensen, once researched the different possible predictors of LBP, and up to 82% of the inhabitants (male and female) of Glostrup, a Copenhagen suburb, were surveyed to determine potential relationships between anthropometric measurements, flexibility/elasticity of the low back and hamstrings, back-muscle strength, and back muscle endurance with the probability of low back troubles during a 1-year period (Biering-Sorensen, Spine, 1984).

The main finding in this study, which received the prestigious 1983 Volvo Award in Clinical Science, was that good isometric *endurance*, not necessarily strength, of the back muscles (in other words, an ability of the low-back muscles to maintain moderate levels of force for prolonged periods of time without significant fatigue) was apparently the best preventer of low back trouble in men and women.

Isometric endurance of the back muscles was evaluated by determining how many seconds an individual was able to keep the unsupported upper part of the body (from the superior border of the hip bones) horizontal while lying prone (tummy down) with arms folded across the chest and the buttocks and legs fastened to a table with wide canvas straps.

In a subsequent investigation carried out in Helsinki, Finland and reported in Clin Biomech 1995, spinal physical capacity and static back endurance testing were again studied for their ability to predict the first-time occurrence of back injury.

Of a total of 126 individuals who were completely free from back problems at the beginning of the research, 33 individuals developed low back maladies over a 1-year period. As it turned out, the results of a static back endurance test (again, a test of the ability of the back muscles to generate moderate force for extended periods) were the only measurement that indicated an increased risk of low back injury. In fact, individuals with poor back muscle endurance were more than three times more likely to develop back troubles, compared with individuals with regular, medium endurance.

In these studies, age/sex/occupation and muscular-strength tests (repetitive sit-ups, arch-ups, squats, and lifts) were all reviewed as possible candidates for low back pain prediction, but only the Volvo examination best predicts LBP. In fact, for both men and women who were unable to maintain the Volvo test for more than 58 s were the most likely to have agonizing spinal problems during the 1-year period. For details concerning the often used trunk performance test in Scandinavian countries, the reader is referred to the article by Alaranta et al. (Scand J Rehabil Med, 1994). An example of the hardware needed in the performance of the test is illustrated in Fig. 24.

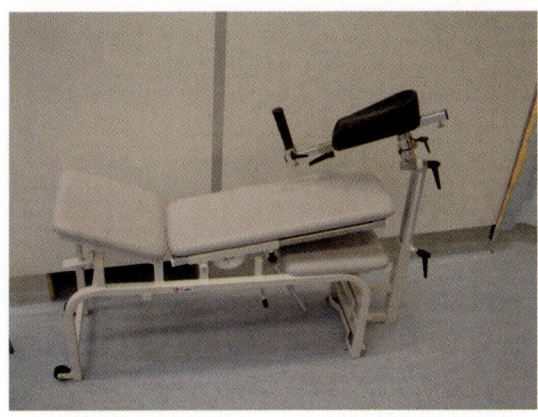

Fig. 24 Hardware used to test for static back endurance or the Volvo examination

Having said that, a recent research paper from the Netherlands tries to proclaim and cast doubts on conclusions reached by the famous award-winning study by Biering-Sorensen (Spine, 1984), the author mentioned that some of the studies that claim that back endurance power is the key have limitations in research quality, particularly the paper by Luoto et al. (Clin Biomech, 1995). Despite these comments, the author is positive that many other orthopedic surgeons and peers still believe that static back endurance testing is a good objective predictor of future LBP as some of the findings of the original famous study by Biering-Sorensen were reproduced by subsequent investigators reaching the same conclusion as published in the journal *Clinical Biomechanics*.

Present Case Scenario

In the present case scenario, the jockey was tested using the original testing criteria as reported by Sorensen, with the help of the hardware as depicted in Fig. 24. It turned out that Johnathan has very good back endurance, and Johnathan subsequently left your clinic a very happy man with a grin on his face.

Learning Point

- A previous award-winning scientific paper showed that for both men and women, those who were unable to maintain the "Volvo test" for more than 58 s were the most likely to have agonizing spinal problems during the 1-year period. For details concerning the often-used trunk performance test in Scandinavian countries, the reader can refer to the article by Alaranta et al. (Scand J Rehabil Med, 1994).

- A recent paper in Pain 2007 confirms that there is no evidence that trunk muscle strength per se has predictive value. The doubts cast by the same paper on the Volvo award winning paper probably need to be taken with a pinch of salt as the magic 58 s was reproducible in other studies subsequent to that by Biering-Sorensen, the Danish spine specialist.

- An emerging potential new prognostic indicator, however, of predicting back pain involves the bedside testing of the transversus abdominis and multifidus muscle by the prone "abdominal drawing-in" test with or without the help of ultrasound and/or bedside EMG (Jull et al., Aust J Physiother, 1993). This point will be further discussed elsewhere in this book.

References

1. Biering-Sorensen F (1984) Physical measurements as risk indicators for low back trouble over a one-year period. Spine, 9:106–19 [The Volvo Award in Clinical Science]
2. Biering-Sorensen F, Thomsen CE, et al. (1989) Risk indicators for low back trouble. Scand J Rehabil Med, 21:151–7
3. Luoto S, Alaranta H, et al. (1995) Static back endurance and the risk of low back pain. Clin Biomech, 10:323–4
4. Hamberg-van Reetten HH, Blatter BM, et al. (2007) A systematic review of the relation between physical capacity and future low back and neck/shoulder pain. Pain, 130:93–107

Enthusiasm for "Non-fusion Technology" for Discogenic Back Pain

History and Examination

You were approached by Peter the orthopedic partner of your clinic and a hand surgeon. He seeks your opinion of whether to proceed with the much popularized lumbar disc replacement for his close friend, 40-year-old Jacky, who has discogenic back pain arising from a degenerate lumbar L4/5 inter-vertebral disc with positive discogram only at L4/5 with reproduction of concordant symptoms and corresponding clinical presentation. Jacky is a physiotherapist, and has read exhaustively on the internet about this emerging popular technology, some implants of which like ProDisc are now being FDA approved. Needless to say, Jacky, by nature of his profession has exhausted the various physical modalities of treatment and exercise therapy but to no avail. You found on the lateral radiograph that Jacky has relatively preserved disc heights for all lumbar motion segments apart from L4/5, although you did find an element of early facet joint degeneration at that level, there was no spondylolisthesis, and the lumbar lordosis was maintained. Would you recommend total disc arthroplasty for Jacky or consider other options? How will you proceed from here?

Discussion

Introduction

In the recent few years, there has been enthusiasm for non-fusion technologies in the management of discogenic LBP as well as some cases of disc prolapse owing to its possible edge over segmental spinal fusion, as the latter is not a motion-preserving procedure and the resultant increased stresses on nearby motion segments can result in adjacent segment disease. Another attraction of lumbar disc arthroplasty is that it is a reconstructive procedure with the hope of reproducing the normal local biomechanics as far as possible. In this respect, it is analogous to the setting of THR and TKR surgeries. Thus, Jacky's preference for non-fusion technology is a fair one, after you ruled out his "early" degenerate facet joints at the same level as the pain generator.

As for implant choice, given a variety of implants to choose from, those implant designs that best reproduce the local biomechanics, are user friendly, and preferably have a good clinical track record will be given priority. In the USA, the two formally FDA-approved implants are the Charité (which our patient preferred) and the ProDisc. The other two models, namely Flexicore and Maverick, are currently under FDA "continuous access" mode.

Rationale of Lumbar Disc Replacement
- To recapitulate, the main rationale of lumbar disc arthroplasty is that it attempts to restore motion, thus producing a more natural and physiologically sound and not a stiffening procedure, but a reconstruction procedure.
- Theoretically, it may avoid adjacent segment premature degeneration as with single segment fusion – but there are no long-term results to confirm this point as yet.
- Although revision is difficult, unless in special cases (e.g., sepsis, dislodgement), it can be revised by posterior fusion.

General Keys to Success
- Need to re-mobilize the disc segment, or else little motion will possible postoperatively and defeats the purpose of the operation.
- However, over-stuffing the joint with an over-sized prosthesis is not advisable either (AAOS 2006 Proceedings).
- Preoperatively, carefully assess the status of the facet joints, to ensure it is not the cause of the pain generator, and the status of the adjacent segments.

- Careful restoration of the sagittal profile, which in the case of the lumbar spine refers to proper restoration of normal lordosis.

Summary of Overall Pros and Cons of Non-fusion Technology

Pros:

- Preserves motion
- Less adjacent segment problem
- Encouraging early results of the ProDisc FDA trial by workers like Delamarter among others (Spine, 2007)
- Spinal fusion has an overall success rate of 80% only; the assessment of fusion with fusion cages is difficult

Cons:

- Problems of reimbursement
- Lack of long-term clinical results; in the USA they are over the 4–5-year mark
- Revision is sometimes difficult and carries morbidity and mortality if the implant gets infected or dislodged whereby the surgeon will sometimes be forced to go in anteriorly rather than resorting to a posterior fusion

General Indications

- Currently, FDA-approved lumbar disc replacement is for a single level only, but there are encouraging early results in some trials that involved multi-level replacements.
- The typical patient is one with recurrence of symptoms after previous discectomy and a lack of advanced facet joint degeneration in the affected spinal motion segment. The disc space is not chronically and severely lost like "bone on bone", but those with discogenic pain with no previous operations, like our patient, can also be candidates.

Contraindications

- Uncertain of the diagnosis or the pain origin
- Already advanced facet degeneration and disc space status, almost "bone on bone"

- Lack of expertise
- Unrealistic expectations of the patient

Current Models
- Semi-constrained: like the FDA-approved ProDisc, on the market since 2004.
- Unconstrained: no FDA-approved unconstrained prosthesis is currently available; there is the possible danger of diminished load share and an increased rate/chance of facet arthrosis of the operated motion segment.

Charité
Biomechanical Rationale
- The Charité was designed to restore disc space height, to restore motion segment flexibility, to prevent disc degeneration at adjacent segments, to reduce or eliminate pain from motion or from nerve compression, and to improve the patient's functional activities.
- It was designed to be biocompatible and durable. It has a life span of 85 million cycles on laboratory testing – more than say THR.
- The Charité Artificial Disc has kinematics that mirror the segmental motion of a normal spine. It is designed to allow anatomic alignment in lordosis, and to allow normal facet joint loading and unloading.
- Wear debris, a concern with polyethylene implants in the peripheral joints, has been studied in the Charité. In a long-term laboratory test of cyclical motion simulating > 11 years of use, no wear debris particles were identified. There is minimal deformation of the core, with less than 8% height loss expected in a simulated 10 years of use.

Implant and Implantation
- The Charité Artificial Disc is a total disc replacement technology that uses two metal alloy endplates and its unique sliding core (Fig. 25). This offers the theoretical advantage of allowing the spacer to shift dynamically within the disc space during spinal motion, moving posteriorly with flexion and anteriorly in lumbar extension. Some

experts feel this may improve the segmental rotation and decrease the possibility of facet impingement at extremes of motion.

- Meticulous attention to implantation is required to ensure that the articulating surfaces of the endplates are parallel in order to restore normal biomechanics. Angled prosthetic endplates are available and were designed to produce parallel surfaces while accommodating lumbar lordosis. Different size endplates are available to the surgeon, so the largest size possible can be used to minimize the chance of subsidence into the bone. Care must be exercised by the surgeon to place the implant centrally in both the sagittal and antero-posterior planes.

- Rotation must be controlled by the surgeon during implantation. The endplates are inserted, and the polyethylene core placed into position as the disc space is distracted. Core dislocation is a rarely reported complication.

- The surgical approach is typically through an anterior retro-peritoneal route. Patient positioning is important so that radiographic confirmation of the implant position can be seen easily by the surgical team. Factors critical for a good result using the Charité are proper patient selection, selecting the correct prosthesis size, and proper prosthesis positioning with the CentreLine Instruments.

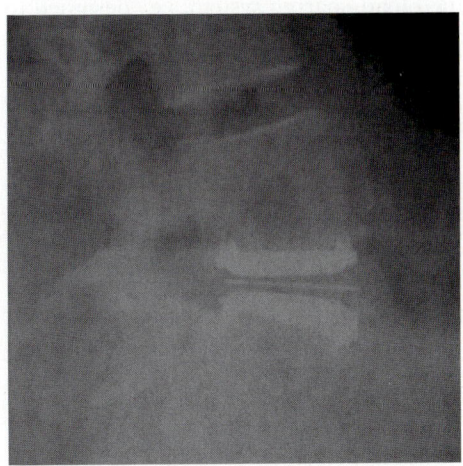

Fig. 25 Lateral radiograph showing a lumbar disc replacement

Clinical Support

- Several clinical studies have been published documenting the European experience with this disc since 1987. Worldwide experience with this unconstrained anatomic disc replacement is now greater than 10,000 cases.

- European experience: clinical results have been reported from Holland (by Zeegers), Italy (by Cinotti), France (by LeMaire), etc., and appeared encouraging, with no reported device failures and around 80% good outcome.

- US experience: The US FDA study was launched at the Texas Back Institute with the first US implantation done in March 2000. Since that time, 294 patients have been enrolled in the FDA multicenter study (196 received the Charité and the rest BAK threaded fusion cages with autografts). The study was completed in December 2001, and the FDA approved the Charité for single-level L4–5 and L5–S1 implantation as of October 2004, and our patient chose to have this implant (Fig. 25).

ProDisc

French Designer and Basic Design

- The ProDisc was designed in the late 1980s by Thierry Marnay. It is essentially a semi-constrained load-sharing system, i.e., designed to have part of the load going through the implant and partly through the facet joints.

- The ProDisc is based on spherical articulations. It has metal endplates made of a cobalt chromium molybdenum alloy (CoCrMo). Physiologically, the ProDisc matches the range of motion in flexion, extension, axial rotation, and lateral bending of a normal spine.

Implant and Implantation

- The convex bearing surface, snap-fit into the inferior end plate, is made of ultra-high molecular weight polyethylene. The artificial disc is attached through a large central keel and two spikes on each endplate.

- The device comes with two endplate sizes, three heights of the polyethylene component and two lordosis angles.

- Minimal access approaches to the lumbar spine, via a retroperitoneal approach, are possible given the design of the instrumentation. Only after the metal endplates are seated in the vertebral bodies is the disc space distracted. The surgeon then check the soft tissue tension, and insert an appropriately-sized polyethylene implant within the disc space, snap-fitting it into the lower metal endplate to complete the assembly process within the body.

US Experience and Clinical Support

- After 8,000 patients in Europe were implanted with ProDisc, the first ProDisc in the United States was implanted at the Texas Back Institute in 2001. Nineteen study centers participated in the prospective randomized study, comparing the ProDisc with the current standard treatment of a 360° front and back fusion using allograft in the intervertebral space and pedicle screws with autograft posteriorly.

- The randomization protocol was 2:1, with two out of every three participants getting a ProDisc and one in three receiving the fusion. ProDisc could be implanted at L3–L4, L4–L5, or at L5–S1. There was also a concurrently running two-level ProDisc replacement study. In the two-level study, patients could be randomized into a 2:1 format if they had two adjacent levels of symptomatic disc disease between L3 and S1. The single-level study arm completed enrollment in April 2003.

- The ProDisc was approved by the US FDA in August 2006 for use at a single vertebral level. ProDisc is the *only* one of the artificial discs undergoing FDA trials that is being investigated for multiple level lumbar disc disease.

Result of FDA Study on Pro-Disc

Delamarter recently reported the result of the FDA-approved ProDisc (Spine 2007), which is a prospective, randomized, multicenter FDA investigational device exemption study of the ProDisc-L total disc replacement versus circumferential fusion for the treatment of one-level degenerative disc disease.

Two hundred and eighty-six patients were treated on protocol at different centers. Patients were evaluated before and after surgery, at

6 weeks, and at 3, 6, 12, 18 and 24 months. Evaluation at each visit included patient self-assessments, physical and neurologic examinations, and radiographic evaluation.

The safety of ProDisc implantation was demonstrated with 0% major complications. At 24 months, 91.8% of investigational and 84.5% of control patients reported improvement in the Oswestry Low Back Pain Disability Questionnaire (Oswestry Disability Index) from preoperative levels, and 77.2% of investigational and 64.8% of control patients met the ≥15% Oswestry Disability Index improvement criteria. Overall neurologic success in the investigational group was superior to that of the control group (91.2% investigational and 81.4% control; $p=0.0341$). At the 6-week and 3-month follow-up time points, the ProDisc patients recorded SF-36 Health Survey scores significantly higher than the control group ($p=0.018$, $p=0.0036$ respectively). The visual analogue scale pain assessment showed statistically significant improvement from preoperative levels regardless of treatment ($p < 0.0001$). Visual analogue scale patient satisfaction at 24 months showed a statistically significant difference, favoring investigational patients over the control group ($p=0.015$). Radiographic range of motion was maintained within a normal functional range in 93.7% of the investigational patients and averaged 7.7° (Spine, 2007).

Other Models
Flexicore

FlexiCore is a metal-on-metal device that is inserted as a single unit. The superior and inferior portions are linked by a captured ball-and-socket joint. The FlexiCore can be implanted from a straight anterior or an antero-lateral direction, and offers the ability to manipulate the position of the implant within the intervertebral space. Unique domed base-plate surfaces are shaped to approximate the concavities of the vertebral body endplates, and are coated with titanium plasma spray to assist bone on-growth fixation. In the US FDA IDE study, FlexiCore was randomized to an anterior-posterior fusion with anterior bone graft and postero-lateral fusion using pedicle screws. Patients with single-level disc disease were studied. The randomized study has been completed, and Flexicore is now in Continued Access mode.

Maverick

The Maverick is a two-piece metal-on-metal design that incorporates a more posterior center of rotation. Maverick began a multicenter clinical trial in the United States in the spring of 2003. Maverick is randomized to an anterior fusion using rectangular LT cages with BMP sponges. The US FDA study is now in continued access mode, the randomized portion having been completed. Maverick is currently being utilized in Europe where clinical series are now also being studied, with large numbers of implantations having been performed in Europe.

Learning Point

- Given encouraging clinical reports on the FDA-approved ProDisc among other clinical data, the question that remains is not only whether lumbar disc arthroplasty will in time become a gold standard treatment option for conditions that are currently treated by spinal fusion in the US, but also cost concerns and insurance re-imbursement issues.
- In the author's view, one significant complication to avoid, just like hip and knee arthroplasties, is infection. This is because while some complications like subsidence may be managed by a more straightforward posterior fusion, in the face of prosthesis infection, removal of the infected prosthesis and attempted fusion in the midst of adhesions is not without risks.

References

1. Zigler J, Delamarter R, et al. (2007) Results of the prospective, randomized, multicenter Food and Drug Administration investigational device exemption study of the ProDisc-L total disc replacement versus circumferential fusion for the treatment of 1-level degenerative disc disease. Spine, 32(11):1155–62; discussion 1163

Extra Busy Banker Troubled by Subacute Back Pain, Yet No Time for Physiotherapy

History and Examination

You have been managing the back pain of the CEO of a local commercial bank Franklin, an extra busy businessman who, despite being your friend, always tells you that he can afford only 2 min of his time for you to speak to him whenever he calls at your office. In the past, Franklin had all the relevant investigations, including a negative MRI of the lumbar spine. You diagnosed non-specific back pain, but, as expected, he is too busy to attend the physiotherapy sessions you recommended. After a recent careful physical examination, you noted suboptimal contraction of particularly his lower transversus abdominis muscle of the lowermost three motion segments with their corresponding multifidus on very careful palpation. You decided to have a senior physiotherapist teach him segmental lumbar stabilization exercises, knowing very well our therapist would be given at most 10–15 min to do the job. How would you proceed from there, as he will be flying to another state early next week in his private plane?

Discussion

There are three systems that contribute to active spinal stabilization according to Panjabi (Spinal Disord, 1992; Curr Orthop, 1994): Passive subsystem (spinal column: bony and capsulo-ligamentous structures), active subsystem (spinal muscles) and neural control.

The active subsystem (muscles) can be divided into two main categories:

- Global, e.g., major trunk movers
- Local: as the name implies, contributes to segmental stability of each spinal motion segment

In this connection, previous researchers have worked out that the most important include the transversus abdominis, and its corresponding segmental multifidus muscle. These two in turn work closely with the diaphragm, as well as the pelvic floor muscles to control the level of intra-abdominal pressure, which in fact also contributes to the stability of the lumbar spine. To realize the importance of the muscular system, the reader should remember that the osseo-ligamentous spine is a long column and inherently unstable, thus subject to buckling (Euler's law), and that in vivo the column requires a combination of muscle forces and muscle stiffness for stabilization (Gardner-Morse et al., J Orthop Res, 1995).

It is a well-known fact that the pathogenesis of as much as 80% of LBP cases is occult. But many now believe that somehow these conditions originate from deviation of the so-called "neutral zone". Neutral zone is a concept introduced by Panjabi (Spinal Disord, 1992; Curr Orthop, 1994). Panjabi's hypothesis identifies control of inter-segmental motion around the neutral zone as a major parameter of spinal instability involved in the concept of clinical stability. When motion occurs in the region of the neutral zone, there is minimal internal resistance, with the ligamentous structures providing restraint in the elastic zone to limit end range of motion.

As a result of the above concepts, the author usually will incorporate thorough postural training after instructing the therapist to find out the best posture that most closely approximates the neutral zone for a particular individual – i.e., this posture may vary somewhat between individuals and not every patient is the same. Notice that the "neutral zone" concept was supported by works by McGill and Cholewicki: namely, that increases in aberrant or uncontrolled neutral zone motion can be countered by increases in activity of the local muscle system.

"Clinical instability" is said to occur if there is a significant decrease in the capacity of the stabilizing system of the spine to maintain the inter-vertebral neutral zones within physiological limits, which results in pain and disability.

Another main theme besides posture is re-training of "local muscles," especially of the last few motion segments of the lumbar spine. This is based on the fact that these (local) muscles could be dysfunctional in many back pain patients. The local muscles may not be able to maintain prolonged or sustained muscle contraction in order to protect continuously any unstable spinal segments, leaving the back pain patient vulnerable to persistent strain and pain. Recent studies also showed that segmental control by the deep local muscle system for spinal support has been linked to both high- and low-load functional activities – a problem in the neuromuscular control of the local muscles by the nervous system has been suggested.

In addition, a very important piece of research in pigs (Spine, 2006) recently revealed that the multifidus cross-sectional area is reduced in acute and chronic low back pain. Although chronic changes are widespread, acute changes at one segment can frequently be identified within *days* of injury. In the past, it was uncertain whether changes precede or follow injury, or what the mechanism was. But these research data resolved the controversy that the multifidus cross-sectional area reduces rapidly after lumbar injury. Such changes are likely due to disuse following reflex inhibitory mechanisms.

The results of this study confirm, for the first time, that atrophy of the multifidus progresses rapidly after injury to a lumbar segment, thus resolving this controversial question. Furthermore, the data confirm that changes in the cross-sectional area following disc lesion are confined to a single segment and have a different distribution to the changes following denervation. These changes were associated with rapid regional changes in muscle histology and chemistry, including enlargement of adipose cells, myofibril clustering, and reduced muscle water and lactate concentration.

The current study provides evidence that rapid changes in the lumbar multifidus occur after injury to a lumbar intervertebral disc, which may be due to disuse following reflex inhibitory mechanisms. Such segmental changes in clinical practice are observed in many back pain patients, not necessarily those with disc prolapse, just like our patient.

But what about the transversus abdominis muscle? In normal people, contraction of the transversus abdominis preceded the onset of contraction of movements involving the upper limb (Hodges et al., Experimental Brain Research, 1997) or lower limb (Hodges et al., Phys Ther, 1997). In other words, there is a *feed-forward* contraction of the transversus abdominis not influenced by the direction of motion of either the upper or the lower extremity. Unlike the other two layers of abdominal muscles, the transversus works independently (functionally speaking) as a muscle corset to help confer lumbar spinal stability. The feed-forward function also helps protect the spine from injury before the patient expects to lift heavy objects. In many back pain patients, there is a significant delay in the onset of contraction of the transversus abdominis, sometimes with a loss of the feed-forward activity (Hodges et al., Spine, 2006).

The therapists who work with the author usually use ultrasound as a feedback (subsequently the patient uses a mirror at home as feedback) to train the lower transversus in the prone position by a method described previously by Hodges and colleagues in Australia.

It was previously shown by Hodges that proper activation of the transversus abdominis will also help activate the corresponding lumbar multifidus muscle. Multifidus muscle training can also be monitored by the use of ultrasound in the presence of an experienced therapist.

Re-learning Motor Control via Bio-feedback

In the current instance, ultrasound was used by the therapists to re-train the weakened local multifidus and the lower transversus abdominis at a few clinic visits. The key to success is summarized in Fig. 26: the diagram reminds Franklin that motor re-learning of the local muscles depends on proper mental preparation on the part of the individual (cognition), we de-emphasize the activity of the global muscles while training the local musculature (precision), training is often helped by biofeedback, and success needs constant drills (practice).

Current Case Scenario

Franklin proved to be a very intelligent individual and a fast learner. The initial clinic biofeedback sessions were followed by plenty of exercises at home with Franklin's wife holding onto a mirror acting as a form of feedback. Franklin made lots of progress and was practicing the taught

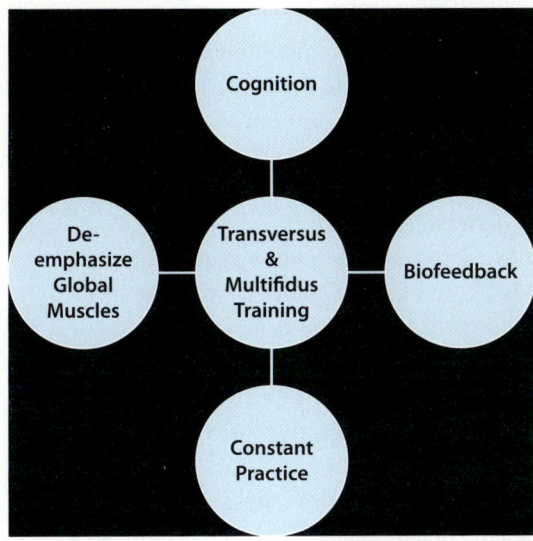

Fig. 26 Four key factors for success in training of local spinal muscle groups: Precision, cognition, biofeedback, and constant practice

exercises whenever free. After he flew back from his business trip, the therapists taught him more advanced functional re-training of the local musculature and proper posture at home based on the basic concepts of neutral zone taught by Panjabi. You met Franklin in the street a couple of days ago and you noticed a grin on his face, telling you that his old friend back pain seems to have left him at last.

Learning Point

- Appreciation of the importance of assessing and re-training the frequently dysfunctional segmental multifidus and transversus abdominis muscle is essential for the success of many therapeutic programs for subacute and sometimes chronic back pain.

- The recent realization that the segmental multifidus can quickly decrease in muscle bulk and cross-sectional area over a short period of time underlines the importance of its re-training, even in some cases of more acute back pain. The underlying mechanism here is likely to be reflex inhibition, rather than one of denervation.

- While endurance is important in predicting future back pain in healthy individuals, in cases of patients with established back pain; the presence of loss of motor control of the local muscles such as transversus abdominis could reflect on the prognosis. In addition, the presence of atrophy of type 1 fibers of multifidus as well as the selective loss of type 2 fibers is also commonly seen.

- It is significant to note that multifidus dysfunction in back pain sufferers tends to persist *even* in athletes receiving an active athletic training regimen or protocol (according to Roy) – which underlies the importance of designing exercise to specifically train up the multifidus and other local lumbar stabilizing musculature.

- The therapeutic exercises described by Paul Hodges' group from Australia is extremely useful in helping to re-train the transversus abdominis and multifidus muscles in LBP patients. Ultrasound is a useful adjunct and may act as a biofeedback device, while the mirror can be used as feedback advice for the patient when he continues the home exercise as taught by the therapists. Biofeedback is a useful method, but success in the re-learning of motor control of these local segmental musculature also depends on cognitive factors, precision factors, and constant practice besides biofeedback.

References

1. Richardson C, Hodges PW, et al. (1999) Therapeutic exercise for spinal segmental stabilization in low back pain. Churchill Livingstone

2. Panjabi MM (1992) The stabilizing system of the spine. I. Function, dysfunction, adaptation, and enhancement. J Spinal Disord, 5:383–389

3. Panjabi MM (1994) Lumbar spine instability: a biomechanical challenge. Curr Orthop, 8:100–105

4. Gardner-Morse M, Stokes IAF, et al. (1995) Role of the muscles in lumbar spine stability in maximum extension efforts. J Orthop Res, 13:802–808

5. Hodges P, Holm AK, et al. (2006) Rapid atrophy of the lumbar multifidus follows experimental disc or nerve root injury. Spine, 31(25):2926–2933

**Metal-on-Metal
Hip Surface Replacement**

History and Examination

Johnny is a 32-year-old real estate salesperson who is very active in different sports like tennis, badminton, swimming, and water-skiing. He was referred to you by his family doctor for left hip symptomatic arthritis. Johnny recalled that 7 years ago, he had on and off aching at the left hip and ever since has been followed up by his family doctor. A previous radiograph of the left hip was done and was passed as normal. He took painkillers on and off and finished several courses of physical therapy sessions from which he found partial relief. Six months ago, his family physician took another radiograph of the left hip since Johnny's pain has deteriorated and detected osteoarthritic changes of the left hip. He was given a further course of physiotherapy and symptomatic treatment since he was told he is much too young for a total hip replacement. However, the pain was not getting any better, and Johnny noticed that the left hip is stiffening up, to the point that he has to forsake all of his favorite sports. As Johnny is determined to resume his previous active life style, he requested his family physician to refer him to you for a second opinion. On examination, the acetabular stress test was positive and there was restriction in the end range of left hip motion in all directions, although the level of pain increases with flexion and adduction. There was no leg length discrepancy, and the old lateral radiograph of the left hip showed the pistol-grip type of deformity. Examination of the lumbar spine and the sacroiliac joints was normal, and there was no neurological deficit. Given the fact that Johnny now has incapacitating pain and stiffness of the degenerate left hip, how would you proceed for further management in this scenario?

Discussion

It is increasingly being realized by hip experts like William Harris that primary osteoarthritis of the hip is at best rare, in fact many patients have subtle hip dysplasia or impingement syndrome as described by Ganz. The former cases may sometimes be amenable to corrective acetabular osteotomies like Ganz's Bernese peri-acetabular osteotomy, while the latter cases may sometimes be amenable to an intra-articular corrective hip procedure thanks to the description of the technique of surgical dislocation of the hip by Prof. Reinhold Ganz.

However, for young patients, especially those in the second or third decade of life who already present to you with arthritis, hip surface replacement helps maintain function, and is frequently compatible with a continued active life-style such as the very sporty individual in this case scenario, a function that is unparalleled by those patients subjected to the standard THR. This is because even in the best hands such as in the Wrightington Hospital's experience, the survivorship of the acetabular component in particular at the 20-year mark in a series of 226 THR for young adults (average age 32 years) is at most around 50% (Sochart and Porter, J Bone Joint Surg Am, 1997). The above underlines the recent trend toward hip surface replacement for young patients with hip arthritis.

Indication for Hip Surface Replacement (According toNICE Guidelines)
- Young and active < 65
- Severe pain and disability
- High demand and high activity level, e.g., high-demand sports
- Strong wish to return to high-impact activities
- Likely to outlive implant in the foreseeable future
- Adequately trained surgeon, and reasonable patient expectations
- Little cost implication

(2002 Guideline of NICE, i.e., National Institute of Clinical Excellence in England)

Contraindications
- Decreased bone mineral density, menopause, advanced age, low activity level

- On chronic steroids
- Deformed hip
- Large bone cysts
- Small or shallow acetabulum
- Short or deformed neck
- Poor head/neck ratio
- Mismatch between the femoral head and acetabulum

Rationale for Doing Surface Replacements
- Investment for the future, good for buying time
- Low complication except femoral neck fracture (up to 5% in some series, higher chance if done for an avascular necrosis [AVN] hip)
- Bone-preserving (conserve anatomy, more natural load transfer, easier revision to primary THR)
- More normal biomechanics, and more physiological loading
- Much lower dislocation rate, since original head size is restored
- Improved ROM, made possible by a large head size
- Less friction since large head with even fluid film lubrication if newer models are used (Fig. 27), low friction implies lower wear
- Ease of revision if the need arises

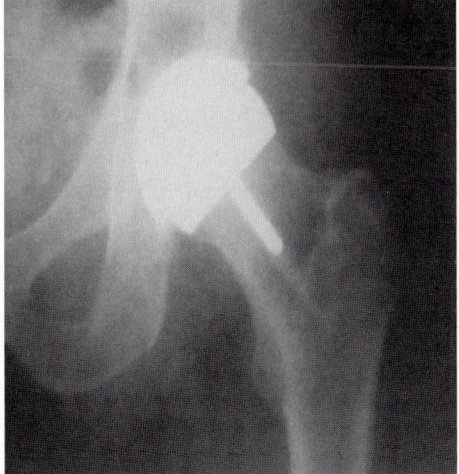

Fig. 27 Patient's postoperative radiograph after left hip metal-on-metal surface replacement

- Shorter rehabilitation time, and functional rehabilitation more easily achieved
- Shorter hospital stay is expected
- Minimally invasive implantation reported and is compatible with this technique (reported by McMinn and Daniel, Proc Inst Mech Eng, 2006) as well as compatible with fluoroscopic navigation systems recently reported in the literature (Belei et al., Comput Aid Surg, 2007)
- Earlier return to work

Quality of Life Issues

In a recent definition of "Health Related Quality of Life" (QOL) Peter Fayers in 2000 commented that QOL should include not only the frequently reported physical functioning, but also social well-being, role functioning, emotional functioning, cognitive functioning, sexual functioning, etc. In the face of tackling an OA hip in a young active patient of reproductive age, hip resurfacing plays a definite role in improving health-related QOL for our patients as opposed to conventional THR. Long-term results are not yet available, but are eagerly awaited.

Newer Generation of Hip Resurfacing Implants

As McMinn and Daniel pointed out (Proc Inst Mech Eng, 2006), hip resurfacing is not a modern concept. Professor Sir John Charnley attempted the first hip resurfacing procedure in the 1950s. This implant failed as a result of unsatisfactory materials and the same problem has troubled hip resurfacing developments over the subsequent 40 years. Modern hip resurfacing using metal-on-metal bearings has shown good medium-term results in the most challenging subgroup of young active patients.

Currently, the latest generation of implant involves metal-on-metal articulation (Fig. 27), instead of a metal-on-polyethylene type of articulation with cemented femoral stem and cementless acetabular component. An example is that marketed by Depuy. Ultimately, however, whichever metal-on-metal implant one wishes to choose, the ultimate performance depends on the metallurgy, the precision of manufacturing, clearance between the head and the socket, and lubrication attained in order to minimize wear and minimize friction to decrease the chance of loosening. The author is aware that not all these details are listed in every hip re-surfacing implant on the market, and it is hoped that more information concerning these aspects will be included in the future.

Learning Point

- As Amstutz pointed out, hip surface arthroplasty has many attractive features for young active patients, particularly because of the conservative nature of this treatment and its ability to preserve femoral bone. It is more anatomic and physiologic than stem-type hip replacements, and it represents a truly *minimally osteoinvasive* procedure, with no penetration into the femoral intramedullary canal. In addition, the construct has increased stability because of the near-normal diameter of the femoral component compared with most conventional hip replacement components.

- In the eyes of the rehabilitation specialist, the procedure can potentially restore the relatively *active life-style* of these young individuals, including participating in high-impact activities, and the much lower dislocation rate lessens the stringent requirement of traditional joint protection methods to follow after THR. Early results reported from Europe and Japan are encouraging, and the technology is likely to be compatible with an improved quality of life for these young people.

- Whether better surgical techniques like surgical dislocation of the hip, or the use of the newly described computer-aided hip surface replacement have added advantage in reducing significant complications such as femoral neck fracture remains to be seen.

References

1. McMinn D, Daniel J (2006) History and modern concepts in surface replacement. Proc Inst Mech Eng [H], 220(2):239–51
2. Belei P, Skwara A, et al. (2007) Fluoroscopic navigation system for hip surface replacements. Comput Aid Surg, 12(3):160–7
3. Sochart DH, Porter ML (1997) The long-term results of Charnley's low-friction arthroplasty in young patients having degenerative arthrosis, congenital dislocation, and rheumatoid arthritis. J Bone Joint Surg Am, 79(11):1599–617

A Young Lady with AVN after SARS

History and Examination

You received a referral from a chest physician who has been dealing with the respiratory sequelae of the SARS virus in a 32-year-old lady, Mrs Smith, who complained of dyspnea and diffuse musculo-skeletal aches and pains, which are most severe around the left knee. Mrs Smith contracted the SARS virus 1 year ago while in Asia, had severe pneumonitis that responded to high-dose steroids. There was bilateral hip and knee pain during her stay in the acute medical ward, and MRI of both hips and knees only revealed "non-specific subchondral anomalies" of both knees, but no mention of avascular necrotic patches at the femoral head or around the knees was made. Repeat MRI of both knees were done last month when she flew back to the USA in view of increasing symptoms of the left knee and showed segmental AVN at the left femoral condyle. What is your plan for management?

Discussion

Introduction

The SARS epidemic in 2003 resulted in more than 8,400 SARS cases and approximately 800 deaths worldwide. Existing in non-identified animal reservoirs, SARS-CoV continues to represent a threat to humans although more than 4 years have passed since a large outbreak of SARS, and no new cases have been reported. However, we cannot exclude the possibility of a re-emergence of SARS. It is hence necessary to understand the biology of the SARS-CoV to deal adequately with the next outbreak whenever it happens, including orthopedic aspects as practicing orthopedic surgeons.

The complete genetic sequence of the SARS virus is now available. The sequence has also been BLASTed. There are some groups who have asked whether the SARS virus was the result of genetic engineering, but this is pure conjecture at best pending further investigation; however, if recombination played a role in the origin of the SARS virus, this would theoretically show up in its sequence.

RT-PCR is a quick, easy, and convenient way to detect the virus. RT-PCR involves real-time reverse transcription-polymer chain reaction assays.

The SARS-CoV represents a novel coronavirus with a large (approximately 30,000 nucleotides) positive-sense, single-stranded RNA containing 14 functional open reading frames (ORFs) of which two large ORFs constitute the replicase gene that encodes proteins required for viral RNA syntheses. The remaining 12 ORFs encode the four structural proteins: spike, membrane, nucleocapsid, and envelope; and eight accessory proteins. The viral genome and its expression within the host cell undergo extensive translational and enzymatic processing to form the 4 structural, 8 accessory and 16 non-structural proteins (Satija and Lal, Ann N Y Acad Sci, 2007).

Common Orthopedic Symptoms after SARS

- Fibromyalgia-like symptoms (Tian et al., Chin Med J, 2006).
- Joint pain was common after SARS infection, but was not a useful clinical indicator of osteonecrosis (Radiology, 2005).
- PFJ (patello-femoral joint) symptoms are not uncommon.
- Non-specific generalized numbness and weakness are present.
- Besides pain in the joint, bone pain is also very common and in some patients is rather persistent and of a dull, nagging nature. Associated MRI and X-ray changes are not always present, although not uncommonly, MRI reports carry comments like "non-specific marrow and/ or subchondral changes".
- Avascular necrosis: commonly of the hip, but occasionally around the knee as in this lady (Fig. 28). AVN may be due to the high doses

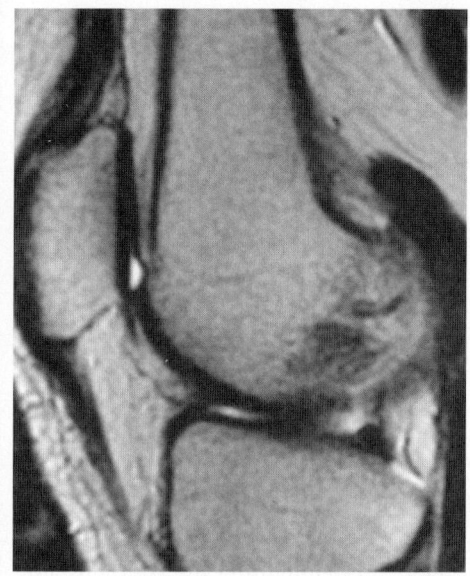

Fig. 28 Sagittal cut MRI showing avascular necrosis changes in the left distal femur

of steroids, but some believe the virus itself may predispose to AVN changes, although this is not yet proven beyond doubt.

Radiological Assessment

In a recent study from Hong Kong, although 53% out of a total of 254 patients had recent onset of large joint pain, 211 out of 264 painful joints (80%) were *not* associated with abnormality on MR images. MR images in 12 out of 254 patients (5%) showed evidence of "subchondral osteonecrosis" in the proximal femur ($n=9$), distal femur ($n=2$), and proximal and distal femora and proximal tibiae ($n=1$). Additional non-specific subchondral and "intramedullary bone marrow abnormalities" were present in 77 out of 254 patients (30%; Griffith et al., Radiology, 2005).

Relation Between Steroid Dose and AVN

- Results of multiple logistic regression analysis confirmed cumulative prednisolone-equivalent dose to be the most important risk factor for osteonecrosis.
- The risk of osteonecrosis was 0.6% for patients receiving a less than 3 g and 13% for patients receiving a more than 3 g prednisolone-equivalent dose (Radiology, 2005).

Management

- Prevention: Recently, researchers attempted identification of essential genes as a strategy to select a SARS candidate vaccine using a SARS-CoV infectious cDNA (Almazain et al., Adv Exp Med Biol, 2006), and a separate group claimed success in inducing high levels of neutralizing antibodies in monkeys (Qin et al., Vaccine, 2006). Whichever method is used, the vaccine should be able to induce immune responses specific to SARS CoV.
- Sharing of epidemiological data and maintaining the GenBank nucleic acid sequence database (nucleic acid research, 2004) is most important.
- Acute and prompt management of the acute respiratory failure not infrequently with ventilator support is required.
- AVN management: is along conventional lines as described by a companion textbook by the author. It is unresolved whether each and every AVN cases post-SARS are necessarily due to steroids, since there are some researchers who suspect that AVN might sometimes be caused by the SARS virus itself.

Present Case Scenario

Surgery in the form of decompression was offered but declined by Mrs Smith. You resorted to the use of pulsed electromagnetic field therapy with some degree of success. Furthermore, Mrs Smith was seen by the psychiatrist of the multi-disciplinary team and treated for depression. You scheduled Mrs Smith for periodic radiographic checks lest there is bony collapse, as a result of creeping substitution; a follow-up MRI was also booked, scheduled to be performed half a year later.

A Final Word on Pulsed Electromagnetic Fields

Nature of Pulsed Electromagnetic Fields

These are devices that produce low energy (much lower than short-wave diathermy) and time-varying magnetic fields, usually for the purpose of achieving bone healing effects and mainly act on bones; its use in avascular necrosis of the bone has long been reported (Clin Orthop Relat Res, 1989).

Application

These devices have been used mainly in treating non-unions and osteonecrosis. They are applied daily for a few hours each session. The degree of magnetic field strength produced is 1.000–2.000 Gauss.

Examples of Clinical Usage

- Non-unions (Calcif Tissue Int, 1991; Foot Ankle Int, 2004; Clin Orthop Relat Res, 2001)
- Osteonecrosis and Perthes (J Prosthet Orthot, 1997)

Learning Point

- Joint pain in a SARS patient does not necessarily point to AVN.
- Non-specific MRI abnormality like "marrow and subchondral signal changes" are much more common than frank AVN.
- Whether AVN cases post-SARS are all the result of high-dose steroids or whether some are due to the virus itself is an as yet unresolved issue.

References

1. Griffith JF, Antonio GE, et al. (2005) Osteonecrosis of hip and knee in patients with severe acute respiratory syndrome treated with steroids. Radiology, 235(1):168–75

2. Wang Y, Ma WL, et al. (2003) Gene sequence analysis of SARS-associated coronavirus by nested RT-PCR. Di Yi Jun Yi Da Xue Xue Bao, 23(5):421–3

3. Satija N, Lal SK (2007) The molecular biology of SARS coronavirus. Ann NY Acad Sci, 1102:26–38

4. Qin E, Shi H, et al. (2006) Immunogenicity and protective efficacy in monkeys of purified inactivated Vero-cell SARS vaccine. Vaccine, 24(7):1028–34

5. Bassett CA, Lewis-SM, et al. (1989) Effects of pulsed electromagnetic fields on Steinberg ratings of femoral head osteonecrosis. Clin Orthop Relat Res, (246):172–85

An Athlete Going for Anterior Cruciate Ligament Reconstruction with Little Time for Rehabilitation

History and Examination

Your colleague, who is a sports surgeon, referred Jimmy to you for advice. Jimmy is a very active amateur soccer player who has participated in many local matches. Jimmy suffered a left knee ACL rupture 4 weeks ago, and is due for elective ACL reconstruction as the swelling has died down, with full ROM attained, and no effusion. However, Jimmy appeared rather impatient after the 4 weeks of active physiotherapy he had had, and told your colleague that he will agree only to a home-based rehabilitation program without braces after the coming ACL reconstruction. Describe what you think, and what factors are essential for success supposing you really agree to let Jimmy try to pursue a home-based rehabilitation program after the coming surgery.

Discussion

Introduction

Because of health care funding and health policy changes, there is a need to examine the effects of an evolution toward patient-directed (i.e., home-based) rehabilitation programs for many clinical conditions, one of which is ACL reconstruction. In fact, the main theme of this book is tele-rehabilitation, and the use of virtual reality as an adjunct to making more home-based programs feasible, especially in countries that are much less affluent than the US. Ever since the milestone development of an aggressive ACL postoperative program, the evolution to a brace-free home-based program is very much expected. In fact, home-based ACL postoperative rehabilitation programs do have some support in the literature, while the evidence for and against the use of knee braces will also be explored in an evidence-based manner in the ensuing discussion.

Home-based Rehabilitation: Indication

Home-based rehabilitation is sometimes considered for very intelligent, compliant patients who cannot frequently come back for follow-up by the author for various reasons.

Literature on Home-based Rehabilitation

Back in 2005, Grant et al. from Alberta, Canada reported in AJSM of a study consisting of 145 patients (aged 16–59 years) who attended a pre-surgery education class (Grant et al., Am J Sports Med, 2005). Home-based patients attended four physical therapy sessions, and physical therapy-supervised patients attended 17 physical therapy sessions over the first 12 weeks after surgery. All patients followed the same standardized rehabilitation program. Study outcome measures included active-assisted knee flexion and passive knee extension range of motion, knee range of motion during walking, KT computerized arthrometer results, and isokinetic quadriceps and hamstrings strength. Patient outcomes were dichotomized as either clinically acceptable or unacceptable.

The result was that the home-based group had a significantly higher percentage of patients with acceptable flexion and extension range of motion compared with the standard physical therapy group (flexion, 67% vs. 47%; extension, 97% vs. 83%). There were no significant differences between the groups regarding range of motion during walking, ligament laxity, and strength.

The authors concluded that a structured, minimally supervised rehabilitation program was more effective in achieving acceptable knee range of motion in the first 3 months after anterior cruciate ligament reconstruction than a standard physical therapy-based program. The clinical implication is that athletes undergoing non-acute anterior cruciate ligament reconstruction can successfully reach acceptable rehabilitation goals in the first 3 months after surgery with a limited number of purposeful physical therapy education sessions, allowing recreational athletes more flexibility when integrating the necessary postoperative rehabilitation into their daily activities. Similar home-based rehabilitation programs after ACL reconstruction were also reported by Fisher et al. (Clin Orthop, 1998), and similar ideas by DeCarlo and Sell (J Orthop Sports Phys Ther, 1997).

Pearls to Success in Home-based Programs

- There needs to be proper and accurate femoral and tibial tunnels and extra rigid fixation. To this end, the use of computer-aided surgery is useful. In addition, the use of virtual reality-assisted virtual impingement and stability testing may help; this will be discussed in Section II of this book.
- Use of high stiffness fixation, an example is with the Washerloc (> 500 N/mm). Consider the use of a slippage-resistant, stiff, and strong fixation device, and stiff strong fixation at both ends of the tunnel.
- Try rehabilitation without a brace (see discussion below).

Use of Braces after ACL Reconstruction

We know that a functional ACL knee brace is useful for non-operated acute ACL tear patients (Renstrom P et al., Clin J Sports Med, 2005). However, many studies showed no conclusive evidence of an ACL brace after ACL reconstruction, as reported by Risberg et al. (AJSM, 1999), Moller et al. (Knee Surg Sports Traumatol Arthrosc, 2001), etc. In fact, Risberg's paper in AJSM revealed that prolonged brace wear causes quadriceps wasting. In 2007, Wright and Fetzer reported in CORR level 1 evidence that there is *no* evidence of the routine use of ACL knee braces after ACL reconstruction (Wright and Fetzer, Clin Orthop Relat Res, 2007).

In a recent systematic review published in *CORR* in 2007, the authors also concluded after reviewing the current literature that there is no evidence supporting the routine use of functional or rehabilitative bracing in a patient with a reconstructed ACL. In particular, no studies demonstrated clinically important findings of improved range of motion, decreased pain, improved graft stability or decreased complications and re-injuries. There is thus no evidence supporting the routine use of functional or rehabilitative bracing in a patient with a reconstructed ACL patient.

Improving Tunnel Accuracy and Accuracy of Intraoperative Testing in Anterior Cruciate Ligament Reconstruction

To this end, the advent of computer-aided ACL reconstruction surgery (Figs. 29, 30); as well as the more recent use of the Intraoperative Fluoro-based Pre-drilling Virtual Impingement Test, and the Fluoro-Based Image Free Pre- and Post-reconstruction Stability Testing is useful.

On Fixation Stiffness

In an article by Howell and colleagues from University of California at Davis published in *Arthroscopy* in 1999, fixations of the DLSTG (double-looped semi-tendinosus and gracilis graft) to a button vs. anchor, vs. post, (both with and without compaction of bone) were tested in young human femurs (To et al., Arthroscopy, 1999). The stiffness of each fixa-

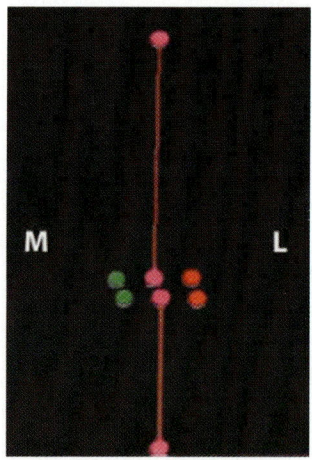

Fig. 29 Computer-aided surgery is becoming popular in various fields of orthopedics besides total joint and trauma, as shown here for anterior cruciate ligament reconstruction

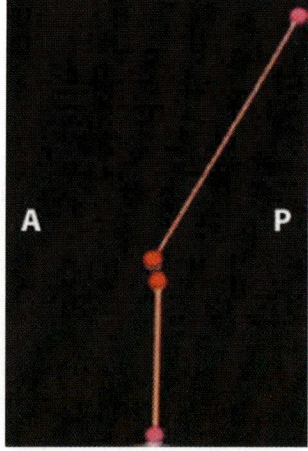

Fig. 30 Besides aiding tunnel placement, newer software is equipped with the capability of performing virtual impingement testing

tion was calculated by modeling the DLSTG graft and fixation method as a series of springs. The stiffness of the femur-button-DLSTG graft complex averaged 23 ± 2 N/mm, the femur-anchor-DLSTG graft complex averaged 25 ± 3 N/mm, and the femur-post with bone graft-DLSTG graft complex averaged 225 ± 23 N/mm. The knot in the suture loop was the least stiff component and determined the stiffness when the DLSTG graft was fixed with both the button and anchor. Compaction of bone significantly increased stiffness by an average of 41 ± 14 N/mm ($p = 0.027$).

Key Message of Howell's Paper

Because the stiffness of femoral fixation methods are 4 to 40 times less than the stiffness of the graft, increasing the stiffness of an ACL replacement would be best achieved by selecting fixation methods with higher stiffness and not by either shortening the graft or increasing the cross-sectional area of the graft. In summary, because the DLSTG graft is stiffer than all the different tested methods of femoral and tibial fixations in this study, the author concludes that the stiffness of ACL reconstruction using DLSTG will be determined mainly by the stiffness of the fixation methods. If a surgeon uses a femoral or tibial fixation method with substantially different stiffness and if the stiffness of both fixations is less than the graft, as is usually the case, then the stiffness of the whole construct will be determined by the fixation methods with the least stiffness, thus underlining the importance of choosing methods of both femoral *and* tibial fixations of adequate stiffness.

Single Vs. Double Bundle

As far as the postoperative rehabilitation program goes, there is some suggestion that the rehabilitation regime after a double-bundle is in fact similar to that after a single bundle (Nau and Sportswood, 2007), but this point is not yet entirely certain at this juncture.

Present Case Scenario

Jimmy eventually underwent elective ACL reconstruction. Postoperatively, he stayed in hospital for 3 days, he was provided with teaching sessions by physiotherapists, together with a VCD summarizing the precautions and home exercises after surgery. He was not given a knee brace. You happened to see Jimmy 12 weeks later in the clinic and KT1000 testing was excellent, the knee range was full, and the patient was satisfied. You also made arrangements for Jimmy to have underwater walking training under the supervision of a trained therapist and he agreed to participate.

Learning Point

- After early aggressive functional rehabilitation being reported in the well-known articles by Shelbourne, in recent years, there has appeared in the literature the use of home-based rehabilitation after elective ACL reconstruction.

- In addition, the latest review on the use of braces also found no solid evidence of the routine use of ACL braces after surgery, as reported in CORR in 2007, assuming properly performed surgery.

- Most authors of rehabilitation texts include excerpts of the protocol they use in their center. But in real life, there are situations in which the patient is reluctant to frequently come back for physiotherapy, either because they live a long distance away, or as in this case is reluctant to come. As a clinician, we still have to find ways to circumvent this problem, and avoid labeling these patient groups as "non-compliant".

- An important article in Arthroscopy found that the stiffness of many common femoral fixation methods is in fact 4 to 40 times less than the stiffness of the graft. Thus, increasing the stiffness of an ACL replacement would be best achieved by selecting fixation methods with greater stiffness and not necessarily by either shortening the graft or increasing the cross-sectional area of the graft. Use of methods of increased fixation stiffness is an important adjunct if a home-based ACL rehabilitation program is to succeed.

References

1. Grant JA, Mohtadi NG, Maitland ME, et al. (2005) Comparison of home versus physical therapy-supervised rehabilitation programs after anterior cruciate ligament reconstruction: a randomized clinical trial. Am J Sports Med, 33(9):1288–97

2. Howell SM, Taylor MA (1996) Brace-free rehabilitation, with early return to activity, for knees reconstructed with a double-looped semitendinosus and gracilis graft. J Bone Joint Surg Am, 78(6):814–25

3. To JT, Howell SM, Hull, et al. (1999) Contributions of femoral fixation methods to the stiffness of anterior cruciate ligament replacements at implantation. Arthroscopy, 15(4):379–87

4. Wright RW, Fetzer GB (2007) Bracing after ACL reconstruction. Clin Orthop Relat Res, 455:162–168

5. DeCarlo MS, Sell KE (1997) The effects of the number and frequency of physical therapy treatments on selected outcomes of treatments in patients with anterior cruciate ligament reconstruction. J Orthop Sports Phys Ther, 26:332–339

6. Fisher DA, Tewes DP, et al. (1998) Home based rehabilitation for anterior cruciate ligament reconstruction. Clin Orthop, 347:94–199

The Office Lady with Neck, Shoulder, Arm, and Back Pain

History and Examination

Betty is a graphic designer working in an advertising company. She presented to your office complaining of acute-on-chronic generalized neck, shoulder, elbow, arm, and back pain after working incessantly for long hours creating 3D images for the potential buyers of different companies. In the past, she has felt similar aches and pains, but the symptoms have definitely worsened lately, together with generalized numbness of both upper limbs so that they keep her from working. As she has been on sick leave for 2 weeks already, being treated by TENS and painkillers by her family doctor, but has failed to improve, Betty was getting worried and has come to your orthopedic service for treatment and advice. How would you proceed from here?

Discussion

Introduction

Most of us are accustomed to encountering patients suffering from neck and back pain after prolonged use of visual-display units such as a computer workstation, as in this graphic designer.

For the back pain, prolonged poor posturing can cause a relatively fixed reversed lumbar lordosis. In these scenarios, simply giving a lumbar pad or support alone, which is very popular nowadays, does not work, and only succeeds in pushing the patient's trunk further down the seat.

As for the neck, many patients and office workers tend to hold their heads in a flexed posture, say 20–30°, this will cause more easy fatigue of the erector spinae muscles at the posterior tension band of the cervical spine, as more force needs to be exerted by the erector spinae muscles to balance the head in this posture instead of sitting with the head erect. The result is easy fatigue, neck pain, and recent studies report that there may even be alteration in muscle activation patterns.

Underlying Etiologic Factors

The causes of this symptom complex with the use of visual-display units are multifactorial and include:

- Physical factors
- Individual factors
- Psychosocial factors
- Ergonomic factors

Commonest Etiology

Prolonged positioning away from the ideal posture will affect neural and other soft tissues in the upper extremity.

Abnormal postures and positions may result in chronic nerve compression or may shorten muscles, and, if the muscle crosses over a nerve, compression may occur. These postures may also contribute to muscle imbalance (Novak, J Orthop Sports Phys, 2004).

Pathomechanics of Commonly Associated Tendinopathies

- Tendinopathy affects millions of people in athletic and occupational settings and is a nemesis for patients and physicians. In Betty's case the arm, shoulder and elbow pain may reflect an element of associated tendinopathies.
- Mechanical loading is a major causative factor for tendinopathy; however, the exact mechanical loading conditions (magnitude, frequency, duration, loading history, or some combinations) that cause tendinopathy are poorly defined.
- Exercise animal model studies indicate that repetitive mechanical loading induces inflammatory and degenerative changes in tendons, but the cellular and molecular mechanisms responsible for such changes are not known.

- Injection animal model studies show that collagenase and inflammatory agents (inflammatory cytokines and prostaglandin E1 and E2) may be involved in tendon inflammation and degeneration; however, whether these molecules are involved in the development of tendinopathy because of mechanical loading remains to be verified.
- Finally, despite improved treatment modalities, the clinical outcome of treatment of tendinopathy is unpredictable, as it is not clear whether a specific modality treats the symptoms or the causes. Research is required to better understand the mechanisms of tendinopathy at the tissue, cellular, and molecular levels, and to develop new scientifically based modalities to treat tendinopathy more effectively (Clin Orthop Relat Res, 2006).

Management of the Current Case Scenario

Since frequently multifactorial, all factors need to be tackled:

- Job analysis and work-place visit was done by an occupational therapist, or a therapist assigned by the employer.
- Patient education on ergonomic factors given, as discussed below.
- Postural correction and re-training performed by physiotherapists, followed by periodic stretching exercises taught to patient to be performed at the work-place.
- Specific physical therapy program to address the multiple levels and designed to rehabilitate the *whole kinetic chain*, detect signs of any nerve compression with confirmation as necessary by nerve conduction testing, and cervico-scapular muscle imbalance corrected in this case by teaching Betty avoidance of holding the scapulae in a protracted position. More difficult cases may even need taping and biofeedback.
- Behavioral modification at home and at work may be necessary (J Orthop Sports Phys Ther, 2004).

Ergonomics for Workers Handling Visual Display Units

There are eight main categories to which we have to pay attention: these include: the display screen, input devices/keyboard and mouse, work desk, seating, footrest, document holder, illumination, and noise.

Summary of Your Practical Ergonomic Advice for this Scenario

After a work-place visit, your occupational therapist comes up with the following recommendations for this lady:

- Use a chair with arm rests at work
- The same chair needs to have a back rest to support the back and help maintain normal lumbar lordosis
- Height of standard table between 25 and 29 inches (63.5–73.66 cm), judging from the build of this patient
- Tilt the computer monitor screen backward 10–20°
- Recommend 40° viewing angle
- Separation distance of eyes from screen 20–26 inches
- Top of screen is at or below eye level
- Add filter to reduce glare for the monitor screen
- Shoulders should be relaxed and comfortable while seated, avoid prolonged protraction of both scapulae
- Elbows should be parallel to the keyboard
- Avoid excessive bending of the head and cervical spine
- Foot rest should be installed
- Keep wrists in neutral position and add wrist supports
- Keep the most frequently used items within easy reach without significant bending or stretching of body parts

Can We Predict Who Gets Work-related Repetitive Strain Injuries?

The predictors positively associated with work-related repetitive strain injuries found in a recent population cohort study involving 2,800 workers include in a recent study:

- Female gender (odds ratio 1.98)
- Some college or university education (odds ratio 1.98)
- Job insecurity (odds ratio 1.76)
- High physical exertion levels (odds ratio 2.00)
- High levels of psychological demands (odds ratio 1.61; Cole et al., Am J Public Health, 2005)

What Can Employers Do to Prevent Musculo-skeletal Complaints Arising from Chronic Use of Visual-display Units?

In some countries, this takes the form of just filling in risk assessment forms. But these methods will frequently *not* lead to recommendations for rectification, let alone follow-up and review.

In the UK, a good example is set by the provision of a web-based intelligent risk assessment and data management package providing on-line employee training and risk assessment. It features e-learning, reporting, stretching exercises, automated e-mail reminders, as well as data management.

Learning Point

- Correct posture is of utmost importance.
- A recent regimen published in Spine (Suni et al., 2006) using the concepts of "neutral zone" maintenance was found by the author to be useful in helping workers that are forced to work for long hours such as the ever-increasing population of computer workers handling visual-display units.
- By the same token, we stress the importance of the concept of finding the best ergonomically sound posture in connection with positioning of the head/neck region, as well as the upper and lower extremities, but especially the former.
- Employer to introduce variability into the work tasks in addition to proper ergonomics (Delisle et al., Ergonomics, 2006).
- In the busy clinic environment, it is suggested that the orthopod use the following eight screening tests for similarly affected individuals: "the overhead lift, overhead work, repetitive reaching, handgrip strength, finger strength, wrist extension strength, fingertip dexterity, and hand and forearm dexterity test" (Reneman et al., J Occup Rehabil, 2005).

- As for the generalized numbness, prolonged positioning away from the ideal posture will affect neural and other soft tissues in the upper extremity. Abnormal postures and positions may result in chronic nerve compression or may shorten muscles and, if the muscle crosses over a nerve, compression may occur. These postures may also contribute to muscle imbalance (Novak, J Orthop Sports Phys Ther, 2004) and should be avoided.

References

1. Suni J, Rinne M, et al. (2006) Control of the lumbar neutral zone decreases low back pain and improves self-evaluated work ability: a 12-month randomized controlled study. Spine, 15; 31(18):E611–20

2. Novak CB (2004) Upper extremity work-related musculoskeletal disorders: a treatment perspective. J Orthop Sports Phys, 10:628–37

3. Delisle A, Lariviere C, et al. (2006) Comparison of three computer workstations offering forearm support: impact on upper limb posture and muscle activation. Ergonomics, 49(2):139–60

History and Examination

After a series of three amateurs who successfully participated in space shuttles reached the headlines of newspapers across the globe, you were approached by Mr Pickering, a 58-year-old multi-billionaire business-man who wishes to follow suit and have a go at a similar flight mission.

However, his family physician requested that he consult an orthope-dic surgeon before the coming space shuttle as regards bone health, as he picked a space shuttle mission that allows him to stay in space longer than his predecessors and seemed to be "value for his money." He came to your office one day and sought your advice. How will you proceed?

Discussion

Effect of a Microgravity Environment on Bone

NASA scientist Edgerton's recent space flight studies suggest that altera-tions that occur during space flights resemble those that occur in SCI (spinal cord injury). He found that control of the motor pool changes in response to changes in weight-bearing activity. Thus, the physiology of the human body adapted to the bipedal gait is that continuous LL load-ing and sensory input are needed for the established oscillatory circuitry and CPG (central pattern generator in the spinal cord) to work.

After exposure to microgravity for 14 days, rhesus monkeys showed adaptations in the tendon force and electromyographic amplitude ratios of different muscles, indicating that their patterns of muscle recruitment were reorganizing, similar to SCI cases. Also, previous NASA studies in astronauts returning from space also revealed rapid loss of bone mass, sometimes up to 30% in 30 days.

Recent animal experiments in mice revealed that reduced mechanical forces in the murine model of unloading by tail suspension increases the prevalence of osteocyte apoptosis, followed by bone resorption and loss of mineral and strength.

Within 3 days of tail suspension, mice exhibited an increased incidence of osteocyte apoptosis in both trabecular and cortical bone. This change was followed 2 weeks later by increased osteoclast number and cortical porosity, reduced trabecular and cortical width, and decreased spinal BMD and vertebral strength. Importantly, whereas in ambulatory animals, apoptotic osteocytes were randomly distributed, in unloaded mice, apoptotic osteocytes were preferentially sequestered in endosteal cortical bone – the site that was subsequently resorbed. The effect of unloading on osteocyte apoptosis and bone resorption was reproduced in transgenic mice in which osteocytes are refractory to glucocorticoid action, indicating that stress-induced hypercortisolemia cannot account for these effects.

The effect or signaling path for the mechanical signals probably involves activation of integrin/cytoskeleton/Src/ERK signaling pathway, and osteocyte survival provides a mechanistic basis for the profound role of mechanical forces, or lack thereof, on skeletal health and disease (Plotkin et al., Am J Physiol Cell Physiol, 2005).

The findings of the recent experiments indicated that diminished mechanical forces eliminate signals that maintain osteocyte viability, thereby leading to apoptosis. Dying osteocytes in turn become the beacons for osteoclast recruitment to the vicinity and the resulting increase in bone resorption and bone loss (Aguirre et al., J Bone Miner Res, 2006).

Effects Besides Altered Bone Health: Orthostatic Hypotension

Recent research showing that astronauts had similar physiological changes to SCI patients in terms of orthostatic hypotension, which can occur in astronauts returning from space, is worthy of note. It is now believed that alterations in nitric oxide metabolism is involved in the pathogenesis of microgravity-induced cardiovascular deconditioning among astronauts returning from space as well as in some SCI cases (Vaziri, J Spinal Cord Med, 2003). For readers interested in other physiological changes in space travel, the review by Payne et al, just published in American Journal of Physical Medicine and Rehabilitation July 2007 is recommended.

Current Case Scenario

Going back to the current case scenario, you advised Mr Pickering, whose DXA turns out to have a T-score of –2.2, against space travel or cut short the travel if he insists on participating. This is because history told us that even well-trained astronauts lose bone mass very quickly in the microgravity environment of space travel, as much as 30% in 1 month in some cases, amongst other possible complications like orthostatic hypotension. A thorough metabolic and cardio-pulmonary check is essential before you will personally endorse space travel for Mr Pickering. You may consider re-training his musculoskeletal system with a full course of hyper-gravity stimulation therapy (as described earlier in this book) upon his return from space and after his vital signs and cardiopulmonary condition stabilize.

Learning Point

- Rapid loss of bone mass and cardiovascular de-conditioning can occur in astronauts returning from space.
- The former is likely due to the absence of periodic weight-bearing mechanical forces involved in the human bi-pedal gait, thereby eliminating signals that maintain osteocyte viability, leading to apoptosis. Altered motor neuron pool firing and the central pattern generator in spinal cord may result, while the latter is likely to be mediated via altered nitric oxide metabolic pathways.

References

1.   Aguirre JI, Plotkin LI, et al. (2006) Osteocyte apoptosis is induced by weightlessness in mice and precedes osteoclast recruitment and bone loss. J Bone Miner Res, 21(4):605–15

2.   Vaziri ND (2003) Nitric oxide in micro-gravity induced orthostatic intolerance: relevance to spinal cord injury. J Spinal Cord Med, 26(1):5–11

3.   Plotkin LI, Mathov I, et al. (2005) Mechanical stimulation prevents osteocyte apoptosis: requirement of integrins, Src kinases, and ERKs. Am J Physiol Cell Physiol, 289(3):C633–43

4.   Payne MWC, Williams DR et al (2007) Space Flight Rehabilitation. Am J Phys Med Rehabil, 86:7; 583–591

History and Examination

You were attending the pediatric orthopedic clinic the other day, and you saw Peter, who is a 12-year-old boy with diplegic cerebral palsy. He was diagnosed to have crouch gait in another medical center by clinical examination and gait analysis. Peter received physiotherapy and casting, followed by elective surgery at age 8 with bilateral percutaneous tendo-achilles lengthening, percutaneous hip adductor releases, medial hamstring lengthening, and rectus femoris recessions.

With increasing age, Peter's mother noticed his gait to be deteriorating, with an increase in the degree of crouching, pain in the knees, easy fatigue, and now the endurance was only slightly more than one block with a rollator. Peter's GMFCS level deteriorated from level 2 to at most level 3.

On examination, Peter has obvious crouching, the popliteal angles were 60 and 55° on the right and left leg. There was dynamic hip flexion contractures of 15° on both sides, and knee extension was −22 and −20° on the right and left knees respectively. Detailed documentation of physical findings is essential and was reported on a form as illustrated (Fig. 31). How would you proceed to tackle the functional deterioration and increasing crouch of Peter's gait?

	R.O.M			STRENGTH		COMMENTS
	R	L		R	L	
HIP:						
Flexion						
Extension (Thomas Test)						
Abduction (hip ext/knee flex)						
Abduction (hip ext/knee ext)						
Adduction						
Internal Rotation (prone)						
External Rotation (prone)						
Anteversion						
KNEE:						
Flexion						
Extension						
Popliteal angel						
SLR						
ANKLE:						
Dorsiflexion (knee flexed)						
Dorsiflexion (knee extended)						
Plantarflexion						
HINDFOOT:						
Inversion						
Eversion						
FOREFOOT:						
Supination						
Pronation						
Duncan Ely Test (Fast)						
Tibial Torsion						
Leg Length (cm)						
Ankle Clonus						
Selective Control:						
Central balance:						
Spasticity:						

◄ **Fig. 31** Standard forms to objectively chart the result of physical examination before and after surgery for children with cerebral palsy

Discussion

Peter's Functional Problems
You called a multi-disciplinary team to assess Peter and the team identified the following main functional problems including: weak triceps surae, crouch gait with excessive stance phase knee flexion with increased dorsiflexion in stance, limited dynamic knee ROM, and diminished pelvic tilt.

Management Plan
You ordered a gait analysis and found the following in the kinematics profile (Fig. 32):

- Increased stance phase hip flexion
- Persistent knee flexion > 30° throughout stance
- Excessive dorsiflexion throughout stance

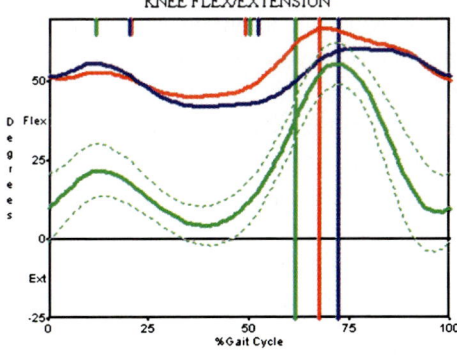

Fig. 32 Notice in the sagittal kinematics profile persistent knee flexion > 30° throughout stance

Likely Pathomechanics from Combined Gait Analysis and Clinical Examination in this Patient

- Tight ankle plantar flexors/increasing height and weight with the adolescent growth spurt
- Overactive knee flexors (with or without rectus co-spasticity)
- Overactive hip flexors
- The plan is to go for multi-level surgery

Main Treatment Principles Before We Embark on Multi-level Surgery

- We need to address all three levels (hip, knee, and ankle levels)
- Preoperatively, you ordered passive stretching by therapists
- Orthoses was initially considered, but finally anterior ground reaction force AFO was not given in view of the high popliteal angle
- Then, proceed to multi-level surgery

Common Surgical Options in Dealing with Crouching

Iliopsoas Recession for Hip Contractures

- Most of the patients selected for this procedure are unable to stand up straight.
- Most have hip FFC (frontal femoral component) of > 30° (on Thomas's test) with or without positive Staheli.
- Kinematics: Typically with two bumps (increased pelvic tilt), decreased hip extension in terminal stance, and increased pelvic tilt in stance.
- Kinetics: Increased internal hip extension moment in mid-stance; GRF falls in front of hip, delayed cross-over from internal extension to flexion moment in mid-stance.
- Role of EUA: Helps differentiate dynamic vs. myostatic.
- Nowadays, the tendency is to lengthen at the pelvic brim level, using the interval between the sartorius and iliacus.

Role of Proximal Femoral Rotational Osteotomy

- Most cases selected for this procedure have in-toeing gait, knees knocking, and tripping.

- Increased femoral anteversion clinically (e.g., by the trochanteric prominence test) should be confirmed with CT prior to surgical intervention.
- CT (2D or 3D) helps define the anatomy of the proximal femur.
- Degree of femoral anteversion calculated using the femoral neck axis and distal femoral condyle.
- Gait analysis: Increased internal rotation (IR) of the hip throughout the gait cycle is often present; the patient tends to internally rotate the hip and tries to minimize the effect of moment arm dysfunction.
- Most surgeons perform the osteotomy at the proximal femur level since it is more precise than a more distal osteotomy. After the proximal femur is osteotomized, the distal segment is rotated externally, and implant fixation is usually by 4.5 DCP.

Tackling Medial Hamstring Tightness
- Tightness of the hamstrings causes difficulty for the rapidly growing child to stand up straight, and walks with the knees bent.
- Knee pain and fatigue with prolonged walking can occur.
- The popliteal angle is abnormal, as in this patient.
- Lateral X-ray of the knee may reveal patella alta, due to overloading.
- Gait analysis: Kinematics profile reveals increased knee flexion at initial contact, with variable knee alignment in the mid and terminal stance, and decreased knee extension at terminal swing.
- Kinetics: Increased internal extension moment through stance, GRF falling behind the knee.
- Dynamic EMG: May show prolonged activation of medial hamstrings in mid stance.
- EUA on table: We need to palpate both the medial and lateral hamstrings.
- Pearl: Lateral hamstring is seldom lengthened unless there is severe crouching or it may result in knee recurvatum.
- Operative procedure in this child: proximal tenodesis relaxes the semi-tendinosus; the distal semi-tendinosus is left free. Concomitant fractional lengthening of semi-membranosus and gracilis is also performed.

Tight Triceps Surae

- Concomitant tight triceps surae usually present as tiptoeing, toe drag, and in-toeing; with diminished ankle dorsiflexion.
- During clinical examination, one tries to determine whether both the gastrocnemius and the soleus are tight by flexing the knee to relax the gastrocnemius in order to isolate the soleus, and look for clonus on fast stretch.
- X-ray: May show foot segmental malalignment, e.g., planovalgus.
- Kinematics: Sagittal plane kinematics on gait analysis reveals plantarflexion in stance and swing, with disruption of the 1st, 2nd, and 3rd rockers.
- Kinetics: Increased internal plantarflexion moment in mid stance (double bump), absent internal dorsiflexion moment in loading response. Decreased internal plantarflexion moment in terminal stance. Premature power generation in mid stance. Diminished power generation in terminal stance.
- Dynamic EMG: Premature activity in terminal swing, premature activity in loading response.
- Concept of three zones and selection of type of surgery:
  - Tackling at Zone 1: (i.e., above the myotendinous junction): This selection lengthens the gastrocnemius, and is used for mild and dynamic cases of equines; not for this patient
  - Tackling at Zone 2: (i.e., at the myotendinous junction) – done in most cases, as in this case scenario
  - Tackling at Zone 3: Non-selective since the tendon is lengthened, reserved for cases that require > 15° improvement in dorsiflexion to achieve the ideal passive range

Learning Point

- Doing the corrections at all levels in one go avoids the need for subsequent repeat surgery, a phenomenon referred to as the "birthday syndrome" by Mercer Rang.
- Literature abounds in support of multilevel surgery, and will not be reiterated here, but is included in the references.

- From the rehabilitation specialist point of view, there is a downside to multi-level surgery: Decreased muscle strength and not infrequently the GMFM scores. Studies from Oxford University found that muscle strength return can sometimes take up to 18 months. Parents should be told this and the child should come back for therapy sessions after multi-level surgery. Also of concern to both the surgeon and rehabilitation specialist is that the optimal time to assess outcome should be delayed to 3 years after multilevel surgery (Saraph et al., J Pediatr Orthop, 2005).

- The lateral hamstring is extremely seldom lengthened unless there is severe crouching lest it result in knee recurvatum.

References

1. Norlin R, Tkaczuk H (1985) One-session surgery for correction of lower extremity deformities in children with cerebral palsy. J Pediatr Orthop, 5(2):208–211

2. DeLuca PA, Davis RB, et al. (1997) Alterations in surgical decision making in patients with cerebral palsy based on three-dimensional gait analysis. J Pediatr Orthop, 17(5):608–14

3. Nene AV, Evans GA, et al. (1993) Simultaneous multiple operations for spastic diplegia. Outcome and functional assessment of walking in 18 patients. J Bone Joint Surg Br, 75(3):488–94

CASE 33   Non-healing Diabetes Mellitus Heel Ulcer

History and Examination

The other day, you attended to an 88-year-old gentleman with a history of DM (diabetes mellitus) peripheral neuropathy and early peripheral vascular disease who is mainly wheelchair-bound with a right non-healing heel ulcer of nearly 4 cm, Mr Thompson, with a referral note in his hand written by a physician consulting you for his non-healing ulcer. You found on examination glove and stocking distribution of numbness, diminished popliteal and dorsalis pedis pulses, but the capillary refill is present and there are no trophic skin changes. The ulcer is not infected, and the edges appear normal, with a clean base, albeit not granulating very well. The general condition of the patient is good, and Mr Thompson proved to be a compliant and co-operative patient. He has been having home sugar monitoring all these years and the recent HbA1c result was satisfactory. You found his fasting sugar to be within the normal range, with a reasonably good level of serum albumen and lymphocyte count conductive of reasonable healing potential. The referring physician asks you to do a flap surgery for Mr Thompson; you decided to give a course of conservative treatment before subjecting Mr Thompson to surgery as his wife and relatives are not keen on surgery either. How would you proceed?

Discussion

Diabetic peripheral neuropathy is prevalent among patients who have had diabetes for several years; in fact, some degree of neuropathy is usually present 5 years after diagnosis.

It is the cause of more hospitalizations than all other diabetic complications combined (Vinik, South Med J, 2002). Total costs of handling these difficult cases exceed $37 billion annually in the USA, and it is a leading cause of diabetic foot ulcers and amputations (Levin et al., South Med J, 2002).

Clinical Presentation of Patients

Chronic Pain
Causes inability to sleep or exercise, traditional treatment involves good blood glucose control and painkillers.

Loss of Sensation
Causes inability to drive vehicles, diminished hand dexterity, affects ambulation status and tendency to fall, and may predispose to amputation. Treatment includes attempted sensory re-education, orthotics, diabetic shoes, compensatory strategies for balance problems and falls.

Recurrent Foot Ulcers
Even in specialty foot clinics, recurrence of diabetic foot ulcers is often very high, generally ranging from 25 to 80% per annum. *Self-care* may be the single most important factor in preventing complications in individuals with a high risk of diabetic foot ulceration. Patients and their families must be able to *monitor* the lower extremities to identify signs of disease and precursors to injury.

For Established Foot Ulcerations
Notwithstanding daily dressing changes, management of associated infection if any, and good DM controls, heel ulcers are notoriously difficult to heal. Before resorting to flap surgery, one may attempt, as in this case scenario, not only to resort to methods of pressure relief, but also to the use of monochromatic infrared energy, which the author finds useful (e.g., Anodyne® Therapy Systems, which was cleared by the FDA in 1994), which may serve to decrease pain, improve circulation and thus healing. Adequate nutrition of the patient is obviously essential.

Mechanism of Monochromatic Infrared Energy Systems

By monochromatic, we refer to a single wavelength of light, which in this case is infrared, and is absorbed extremely well by hemoglobin. Energy delivery is 1.6 J/cm²/min with a uniform energy density over 22.5 cm² of pad, and given in pulses of energy at 292 times per second.

Main Mechanism

The method works mainly by rapid release of nitrous oxide (NO) from hemoglobin, which is a powerful vasodilator of arteries and veins, and also reduces platelet aggregation. In addition, NO is a signaling molecule for angiogenesis, and improves vasomotor activity of lymph microvessels. There is some suggestion that NO may act as direct mediator of the analgesic effect of morphine.

The resultant improved circulation carries O_2 and nutrients to nerves improving nerve trans-membrane potential.

Practical Treatment Guide

Guidelines from the manufacturer:

- For neuropathy: 30–45 min – benefits seen at a minimum of 3× per week
- For wounds: apply 20–30 min once per day, covering the therapy pad with a clear plastic barrier, as was used in this patient
- Pain management/edema controls: 15–30 min – use before physiotherapy to increase/reduce pain and increase tolerance of physiotherapy

Home Treatment Available: Home System Model 120

This can be used up to twice a day as guided by a clinician. One advantage is that it is safe to use in the presence of nearby orthopedic implants (Fig. 33).

Precaution: avoid excessive and prolonged use since it may cause superficial burns.

Contraindications

- Pregnancy
- Active malignancy/sepsis

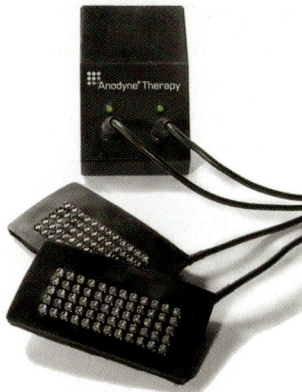

Fig. 33 A home model of a monochromatic infrared machine (Home System Model 120)

Some Literature Support

- Helps restore sensation by monofilament testing and evoked potential response (J Am Podiatr Ass, 2002)
- Improved sensation may reduce falls
- Increased microcirculation, shown by previous studies with laser Doppler, particularly applicable clinically to difficult areas like the *heel* in which even skin flap surgery sometimes fails and breaks down, as in this patient
- Improved wound healing (Adv Wound Care, 1999)
- Reduction in pain and pain medications (Reigger-Krugh et al., J Orthop Sports Phys Ther, 2001)
- Improved quality of life
- Used by many US military hospitals, including Navy Seals

What about Prevention of Ulcers or Recurrence?

- Temperature monitoring instrument to reduce the incidence of foot ulcers in individuals with diabetes who are at a high risk of lower extremity complications.
- Infrared temperature home monitoring, by serving as an "early warning sign," appears to be a simple and useful adjunct in the prevention of diabetic foot ulcerations in a recent randomized trial (Lavery et al., Diabetes Care, 2007).

■ Pilot work in this area suggests that high-risk patients can effectively use an infrared thermometer as a home monitoring tool to identify inflamed tissue and take action to prevent foot ulceration.

(P.S. The thermometer is equipped with a "touch sensor" tip that detects contact with skin. Thus, to operate the device, the user places the tip of the device on the skin, which then automatically triggers a temperature measurement and displays it on a liquid crystal display screen. The thermometer has a gooseneck design, which allows the user to reach any point on the bottom or sides of the foot.)

Learning Point

■ There is an increasing number of rehabilitation specialists, including the author, who propose more and more home monitoring and home-based treatment programs for different orthopedic conditions, such as the Home Model system by Anodyme described here, which appears promising, and the elderly patient with recurrent foot ulceration can receive treatment in the calm atmosphere of his own home.

■ In our present case scenario, home monitoring by infrared thermometer in our patient with a high risk of foot ulcerations as well as home treatment by suitable monochromatic infrared devices under the guidance of a clinician or therapist is likely to be a move in the positive direction as prevention is better than cure.

References

1. Lavery LA, Higgins KR, Lanctot DR, Constantinides GP, Zamorano RG, Armstrong DG, Athanasiou KA, Agrawal CM (2004) Home monitoring of foot skin temperatures to prevent ulceration. Diabetes Care, 27:2642–2647
2. Lavery LA, Higgins KR, et al. (2007) Preventing diabetic foot ulcer recurrence in high risk patients. Diabetes Care, 30:14–20
3. Evidence-based guide to therapeutic physical agents. Belanger, Lippincott (2002)

History and Examination

Patrick is a 43-year-old bartender. He presented to you with subacute onset of cervical radicular pain shooting down both arms, and some numbness of the C6/7 dermatomes on examination, with no objective weakness. There were neither signs of cervical myelopathy nor long tract signs at the lower limb, and there was no sphincter disturbance. A cervical radiograph revealed maintenance of normal lordosis, and was unremarkable except for some decrease in disc space at C6/7, whereas subsequent MRI revealed para-central disc prolapse at C6/7.

A full course of physiotherapy lasting 10 weeks was given with no effect. Patrick has a friend with a similar problem at the C5/6 level who had a cervical disc arthroplasty. When you discussed surgical intervention for his incapacitating symptoms, Patrick revealed a preference for cervical disc arthroplasty over cervical fusion.

Discussion

As far as administration of a new type of surgery is concerned, it is always advisable to first read the guidelines of well-respected institutions instead of jumping in with a new technology prematurely. In addition, it is essential for patients to be aware of the pros and cons of a new procedure before surgery.

One such well-respected institution is "NICE" (National Institute for Clinical Excellence) in the UK.

NICE Guidelines for Cervical Disc Replacement

Following anterior cervical discectomy, a proportion of patients present with progressive spondylosis requiring surgical treatment at adjacent cervical segments. Other possible fusion-related morbidity includes a pseudoarthrosis rate of 15–30%, bone graft donor site problems, 10–30%, hardware-related problems, 1–5%, occasional dysphagia, and overall reoperation rate for cervical disc pathology is 2%.

Reconstruction of a failed intervertebral disc using a functional prosthesis aims to offer the same benefit as decompression, whilst preserving motion at the operated segment, thereby reducing abnormal stresses on adjacent disc levels associated with fusion procedures.

This procedure can be used for patients with acute disc herniation or cervical spondylosis. In these conditions, nerve root or spinal cord compression may cause symptomatic radiculopathy or myelopathy.

Clinical Trials for Cervical Disc Replacement

In two recent randomized control trials with follow-ups of 6 months and 24 months, neck and arm pain scores and quality of life indices all improved after cervical disc arthroplasty. There was no statistically significant difference in outcomes between patients treated with artificial disc implants and those treated by fusion surgery. One case series of 7 patients found significant improvements in arm and neck symptom scores and neck disability index assessment at 6 months, compared with preoperative values.

The largest case series available reported an improvement in clinical evaluation of motor strength and sensory signs, and reported patient self-evaluation of symptoms as "excellent" in 65% of patients having single-level disc replacement (32/49), and 77% of patients having surgery at two levels (20/26).

The range of motion in the treated spinal segment was reported to be well preserved in those studies that included this outcome measure. There were no reported incidents of device failure in 100% of patients (27/27) in the prosthetic disc arm of a randomized control trial, or among 13 patients in a case series. Device migration was noted in 2% of patients undergoing prosthetic cervical disc implant in a case series (2/103), although no migration was greater than 3.5 mm from the initial implant site, and none were associated with neurological symptoms.

In another large case series of patients undergoing prosthetic implants, re-intervention was required in 3% of patients (3/103; 2 patients required treatment for residual symptoms, and 1 patient required evacuation of a hematoma), transient hoarseness in 13% (2/15) of patients, moderate dysphagia in 4% (1/27) and recurrent laryngeal nerve palsy in 4% (1/27).

There are, however, anecdotal reports of heterotopic ossification (Mehren et al., Spine, 2006) and limited movement following this procedure, just as in the case of lumbar disc arthroplasty.

Commonly Used Prostheses

Although there are many cervical disc arthroplasty prostheses in various stages of development, only the two implants with intermediate term outcome data will be mentioned: The Prestige II Cervical Disc replacement, and the Bryan Cervical Disc system.

Prestige II Cervical Disc Replacement

The predecessor of the current implant was the Bristol-Cummins Disc developed by the British neurosurgeon Brian Cummins, as he encountered many problems of adjacent segment degeneration. However, the device proved to be too large for the majority of patients and there were screw breakages and problems with ball and socket mismatch. The refined version Prestige I Disc came into the market in 1998 manufactured by Medtronics, essentially a metal-on-metal construct with articulating surfaces and variable point loading. The lower component, which used to be a hemispherical cup, was replaced by a shallow ellipsoidal saucer permitting translation and 2 mm of freedom in the AP plane. Rotation of the upper component was achieved by allowing the hemisphere of the joint to glide in the saucer. The slightly incongruent interface between the two components of the joint allows the upper vertebral component to passively find its own axis of rotation as determined by the facet joints and coupled motions of the adjacent vertebra.

Further refinements were made to the Prestige II Cervical Disc by reduction in profile, bone ingrowth surfaces, and added size range to adapt to different local anatomies.

The Bryan Cervical Disc Prosthesis

This device from Medtronics consists of a polyurethane nucleus designed to articulate with two titanium alloy surfaces. The bone-articulating surface of each shell includes a titanium porous coating to enhance bone ingrowth and long-term stability. A polyurethane sheath surrounds the nucleus and is attached to the shells forming a closed compartment. Titanium alloy seal plugs provide for retention of a lubricant. Anterior stops on each shell are designed to prevent posterior migration of the device and a means by which the device can be inserted and if needed, removed. It comes in diameters of 14, 15, 16, 17, and 18 mm.

Present Case Scenario

With this in mind, your patient still chose to proceed with cervical disc replacement; the postoperative film is as shown in Fig. 34. He made an uneventful recovery, with no wound infection, hoarseness, dysphagia,

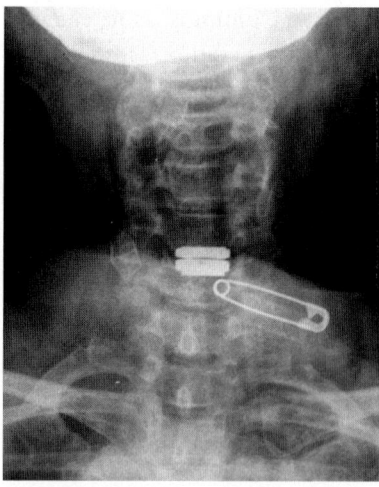

Fig. 34 Postoperative radiograph after cervical disc arthroplasty

etc. During follow-up in the clinic at 4 weeks, you noted a near normal range of motion, the numbness has resolved, and the patient appeared satisfied with the procedure. Overall, the current literature as regards rehabilitation after cervical disc arthroplasty does not differ significantly from that after fusion given the same cervical pathology at hand. Most surgeons feel that earlier mobilization after cervical disc arthroplasty is allowed.

Learning Point

- Ensure that patients understand the long-term uncertainties about the procedure and the alternative treatment options.
- This procedure should only be performed in specialist units where surgery of the cervical spine is regularly undertaken.
- Longer-term data are required to compare the results with those of spinal fusion.
- There are few data available concerning the use of two level (Bi-level) prostheses.
- Little long-term data are available, particularly in relation to potential reduction in adjacent level degeneration compared with fusion – 10-year comparative data may be necessary before efficacy is demonstrated (it takes time for adjacent level degeneration to develop).

References

1. Sekhon LH (2003) Cervical arthroplasty in the management of spondylotic myelopathy. J Spinal Disord Techn, 16(4):307–313
2. Sasso RC. Bryan cervical disc replacement: single-surgeon experience from U.S. IDE. Company abstract. 2004
3. Goffin J, Van Calenbergh F, Van Loon J, Casey A, Kehr P, Liebig K et al. (2003) Intermediate follow-up after treatment of degenerative disc disease with the Bryan cervical disc prosthesis: single-level and bi-level. Spine, 28(24):15

4.   Wigfield CC, Gill SS, Nelson RJ, Metcalf NH, Robertson JT (2002) The new Frenchay artificial cervical joint: Results from a two-year pilot study. Spine, 27(22):15

5.   Porchet F, Metcalf NH (2004) Clinical outcomes with the Prestige II cervical disc: preliminary results from a prospective randomized clinical trial. Neurosurg Focus, 17(3):E6

6.   Mehren C, Suchomel P, et al. (2006) Heterotopic ossification in total cervical artificial disc replacement. Spine, 31(24):2802–6

History and Examination

John is a laborer whose work involves the packing of finished products of a toy company that he works for along with other workers on the assembly line. He is usually seated facing the chair of his workmate, while the assembly line is moving on his right hand side. He comes to your office complaining of diffuse right elbow and forearm pain, acute-on-chronic in onset, with occasional aches in the shoulder and neck area as well.

Physical examination of the elbow by you revealed direct tenderness over the anterior aspect of the lateral epicondyle as well as the postero-inferior aspect. Pain was exacerbated by resisted wrist dorsiflexion, especially with the elbow extended.

The radial-capitellar joint was non-tender on direct palpation and on pronation/supination maneuvers. There were neither signs of postero-lateral rotatory instability of the elbow nor numbness along either forearm. The middle finger test for possible radial tunnel syndrome was negative, and there was no anterior local tenderness along the radial nerve in the interval between the brachio-radialis and brachialis or at the level of the radial neck.

Discussion

Work-related neck and upper limb disorders are common problems among office workers who use computers intensively and maintain prolonged static postures as discussed in Case 30, but similar conditions also occur from repetitive strain of a muscle group, especially coupled with working in awkward positions. The elbow is a particularly vulnerable site owing to the relative imbalance between the large forearm musculature and the small insertion area of the epicondyles of the humerus. The pathomechanics of work-related tendinopathies have been covered in great detail in Case 30 and will not be repeated here.

Initial Assessment

There are altogether eight recommended screening tests that the orthopod or primary care physician can consider using during assessment of the patient in the setting of a busy clinic, viz.: the overhead lift, overhead work, repetitive reaching, handgrip strength, finger strength, wrist extension strength, fingertip dexterity, and a hand and forearm dexterity test (Reneman et al., J Occup Rehabil, 2005).

Rehabilitation Protocol of This Patient

Acute Phase

- Pain relief and inflammatory control – by ice application, electrotherapy (e.g. ultrasound, TENS)
- Mobilization and stretching exercise as tolerated
- Education – knowledge on condition, precaution and care in daily living, ergonomic advice

Subacute and Chronic Phase

- Pain relief – by ice or thermal application, electrotherapy (e.g., ultrasound, short wave diathermy, immunofluorescence technique, self-massage)
- Exercise – continue mobilization and stretching exercise, strengthening exercise to wrist extensor and handgrip as tolerated
- If refractory, proceed to shockwave treatment. The protocol attached (Fig. 35) showed the role of shockwave treatment in the management of subacute and chronic patients with lateral epicondylitis at the author's institution.

Physiotherapy Protocol for Lateral Epicondylitis of AROS service

The recruited patients are divided into 2 groups:
Group1- **Acute unilateral** lateral epicondylitis
Group2- **Chronic unilateral/ bilateral**
        lateral epicondylitis

N.B. Acute: ≤ 6/52 onset
     Chronic: > 6/52 onset

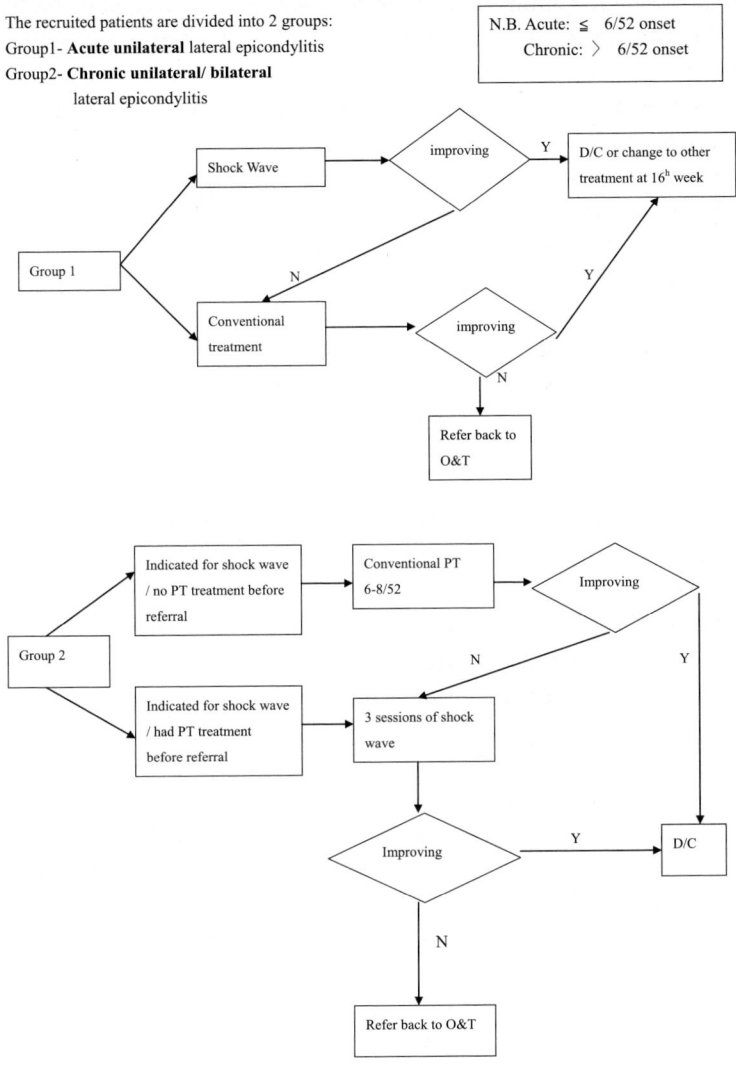

Fig. 35 Workflow in incorporating the use of shockwave therapy for patients with lateral epicondylitis

Use of Shockwave in Lateral Epicondylitis

The protocol, in summary, for the use of shockwave is listed below; the mechanisms of shockwave have been discussed in the companion text already.

- For the resistant group: give two sessions per week for 6 weeks, then review
- For less severe cases or if used as first-line therapy: one session per week for 3 weeks, then review

Ergonomic Advice

Since physical risk factors that contribute to pathogenesis are related to repetition, duration, working in awkward and static positions and forceful movements of the upper extremity and neck, our rehabilitation protocol always involves ergonomic advice given by the occupational therapist.

Outcome Assessment of Lateral Epicondylitis Patients

- Visual Analogue Scale (0–10 scale, both in resting and wrist extension)
- Disability of the Arm, Shoulder, and Hand Questionnaire
- Serial charting of the power grip
- Percentage of overall subjective improvement

Current Case Scenario

In the current case, John's right elbow pain was refractory to conventional physiotherapy measures. He was referred to have shockwave treatment of his right elbow with response. A work site visit was performed by the occupational therapist, with modification of the work routine arranged for John. Then follows a period of work hardening and training in the occupational therapy department of simulated work tasks, before he finally returned to work, given an elbow counter-force brace protection. His employer switched the nature of John's job to one using a visual-display unit computer workstation.

Problems Encountered by Employers in Managing Occupation-related Health Risks and Solution

John's employer expressed the wish to know more about how to document and prevent work-related injuries for both his workers who use visual-display units as well as workers like John who work on the production or assembly line. He has difficulty managing lots of risk assessment records, and in providing systematic follow-up of his injured workers, which has so far led to loss of revenue and work productivity.

Solution Options for Assessing, Recording, and Preventing Work-related Health Risks

- Paper-based risk-assessment check-list – like the one used by the employer is not evidence-based and he wishes for a change
- Hiring a professional risk assessor – deemed too expensive by the current employer
- Computerized risk-assessment system is likely the answer:
  - There is currently an on-line system in the USA to reduce computer-related injuries. In the UK, there is also a complete solution package for Display Screen Equipment providing on-line employee training and risk assessment. Examples of such platforms include: "Workstation Safety Plus".
  - John's employer finally chose a similar system that includes e-learning on the different parts of the work-station, on-line risk assessment, reporting, stretching exercises, automated e-mail reminders, and data management. The new system is also equipped with on-line self-assessment with results automatically fed into a database, and will be channeled to the company's health and safety personnel for follow-up action – another example of how computer systems can be put to good use in the field of orthopedics.
  - As for those workers who remained working on the assembly line, your therapists taught the employer the following guiding principles to prevent injury and promote safety, which are discussed in the next section.

General Basic Ergonomic Principles in Machinery Handling

Principle of Proper Positioning
- Proper positioning of body segments and posture in handling heavy items is important in the prevention of injuries.
- In computer workers, proper arm and wrist supports are particularly important to prevent overuse injuries like elbow lateral epicondylitis, in this case to prevent recurrence of John's lateral epicondylitis.
- For workers with physical impairment or injured workers returning to work, proper periodic counseling and health checks should be provided.

Principle of the Anatomical Control Site
- The control display and command panels of machinery need to be placed in the most comfortable position with due regard to the biomechanics and kinesiology of the human body.
- In workers with physical impairment or injured workers returning to work, the control buttons or control arm of the machinery should be within easy reach of the most functional body part of the patient, always avoid awkward positioning of body parts.
- By the same token, the control panel should be made as simplistic as possible, such as the use of a single switch as opposed to rows of switches.
- Remember that even if the returning worker has fully recovered, work places that have an awkward layout of machines or storage units may make it difficult to use the knowledge of "good body mechanics" taught to the patient by the therapist (Carlton, Am J Occup Ther, 1987).

Principle of Simplicity and Intuitive Operation
- Design of the controls of machinery should be compatible with the intuition of most humans as far as possible, just like closing a valve is by clockwise motion as opposed to a counter-clockwise maneuver.
- These design considerations also serve to minimize errors.

Principle of Notice Suitability

- Notices like warnings or precautions to take should be placed on easily visible parts of the machinery, preferably right next to the control arm or control button to prevent undue hazards.
- For workers with physical impairment such as visual impairment, conveying a warning notice may need use another of the body's senses like use of a siren or sharp warning sound, assuming the hearing of the patient is not impaired.

Principle of Allowance of Recovery from Errors

- Strategies in this respect are many, such as the color-coding of wires, making the machinery or socket connection so that it fits in only one orientation, and prevention of harm to the operator by fusing the electrical appliances.
- For physically impaired workers, with, say, decreased dexterity, then addition of a second set of safety measures like voice commands (e.g., undo connection) will be of help, especially if there is concomitant visual impairment. This will also help prevent undue injury to our patient.

Principle of Adaptability and Flexibility

- Machinery should be made user friendly and easy to handle. This will not only quicken the process of learning, but also lessen the chance of error during busy handling of the machinery. Thus, the importance of a friendly human–machine interface.
- For workers with physical impairments, the device and controls should be made to fit the person, and not the other way round.

Principle of Mental and Chronological Age Appropriateness

- Design of equipment should suit the age of the target group, for instance, rehabilitation equipment for children should preferably have adjustable heights as the child grows.
- In the case of hiring workers with special physical impairments, for instance cerebral palsy and neurodegenerative brain disorders, sometimes they may have a mental age different from their chronological age and corresponding adaptations will be needed.

Learning Point

- The elbow is especially vulnerable to tendonitis owing to the relative imbalance between the large forearm musculature and the *small* insertion area of the epicondyles of the humerus.
- When organizing work for staff whose job nature involves high stresses to the forearm muscle groups, or awkward positions besides repetition, it is important to allow for physical variation with other work tasks, thereby avoiding working with the same task throughout the working day, constant review of the ergonomics of the workplace is part of the responsibility of the employer, although the workers should also participate actively in periodic health assessment for their own good.
- Shockwave therapy can be considered in patients with lateral epicondylitis refractory to conventional physiotherapy.

References

1. Juul-Kristensen B, Jensen C (2005) Self-reported workplace related ergonomic conditions as prognostic factors for musculoskeletal symptoms: the "BIT" follow up study on office workers. Occup Environ Med, 62(3):188–94
2. Szeto GP, et al. (2005) A comparison of symptomatic and asymptomatic office workers performing monotonous keyboard work. I. Neck and shoulder muscle recruitment. Man Ther, 10(4):270–80
3. Decker T, Kuhne B, et al. (2002) Extracorporeal shockwave therapy in epicondylitis humeri radialis. Short-term and intermediate-term results. Orthopade, 31(7):633–6

Chronic LBP in a Laborer Whose Job Requires Repeated Lifting

History and Examination

Simpson works for a small air-conditioning company where his job involves much in the way of lifting objects. He sprained his back at work during one of the lifting maneuvers 3 months ago and has since been on sick leave. Simpson has received both physiotherapy and occupational therapy for the past 3 whole months; both the plain radiograph and MRI of the spine were normal. The good thing about Simpson is that he is a well-motivated hard-working employee who is keen to return to his work. Simpson's employer is eager to have his hard-working staff to return to his work also, but is afraid that Simpson may have re-injury to his back as there are no jobs with "lighter duties" in his small company; thus a functional capacity evaluation (FCE) was arranged by the employer at this juncture. Despite a favorable FCE report, Simpson had very limited work tolerance and is now on sick leave again. Simpson requested his attending orthopod to refer him to you for further rehabilitation of his back problem. Simpson is determined to return to his previous work, and does not want to change his job. His employer also wants to have his beloved staff back as early as possible and is surprised that the preceding FCE report did not fully reflect Simpson's work ability on his attempted return to work. How would you proceed from here?

Discussion

Introduction

Incorrect lifting technique is often responsible for acute pain in the lumbo-pelvic-hip region. Education to have a "safe" lifting technique is important to prevent injury to workers. Forward bending requires flexion of the spine that is in fact controlled by *eccentric* contraction of the erector spinae, multifidus, quadratus lumborum, and extensors of the hip – namely the gluteus maximus and the hamstrings. Prior to this motion, lumbar segmental stabilization and sacral stabilization are needed by the inner or local muscle unit, especially the transversus, multifidus, and pelvic floor muscles.

In addition, the flexibility of the spine is important to maintain, to help reduce the moment arm of the external load by decreasing the distance between the lifted object and the spinal column (Adams and Dolan, 1997).

Subsequent spinal extension is effected by the *concentric* contraction of the gluteus maximus, while load transference through the trunk is maintained by a co-ordinated action of the abdominals and deep spinal stabilizers. The sacroiliac joints, meanwhile, are compressed and stability is maintained through force closure provided by tension in the thoraco-dorsal fascia effected by contraction of the latissimus dorsi, the transversus, multifidus, and gluteus maximus. With the above basic knowledge, you designed a functional rehabilitation program for Simpson.

Functional Rehabilitation Program

The program you designed consists of the following:

- Training of the weakened core or local muscles of the back first, namely the segmental multifidus, and especially the lower transversus abdominis, together with subsequent training of the proper breathing pattern of the diaphragm and pelvic floor muscles to properly control the intra-abdominal pressure during lifting maneuvers – for elaboration of local versus global back muscles, refer to Case 26.
- Afterward, train the global muscles (Fig. 36)
- General aerobic training and psychosocial assessment

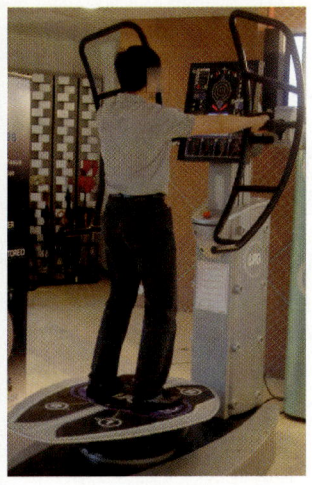

Fig. 36 Commercially available machinery that helps train global core muscles

- Training of the pattern of muscle recruitment specific to the process of lifting, tailored to the nature of Simpson's job:
  - Recruit the core muscles prior to accepting any loading to the vertebral column
  - Keep the load as close to the body as possible near to the center of the base of support of the lower extremity
  - Test the weight of the load prior to actually lifting the weight, get assistance if the load is too heavy, or consider the use of mechanical devices

Key Concept

Many workers may in fact have the weak "link" being located at a time point between the concentric and eccentric contraction of the erector spinae muscle of the back or vice versa. In these situations, specific training of both types of contraction, as well as ways to effect a more proper and smooth transition between concentric and eccentric activity, is required.

Relevant Body Mechanics

- The force required by the erector spinae to balance the body while lifting a load held further away from the body is much higher than if the load is held as near to the trunk as possible given the same weight of the load. This arises because the moment arm is much increased if the load is held further away from the body. Proper patient education is important.

- Similarly, the force on the erector spinae is higher if the laborer chooses to bend at his hips to pick up the load with the knees straight. If the load is not at too low a level, bending the knees allows the upper body to function at a smaller moment arm, and involves less force generation in the erector spinae muscles.

- If the load is small but heavy like some mechanical parts of the air conditioner in this case scenario, it will pay to start in a squatted posture before initiation of the lifting maneuver, as in this patient.

Functional Capacity Evaluation

Functional capacity evaluation (FCE) is measurement of the patient's performance in a comprehensive series of standardized tests, resulting in data that can be interpreted according to the predictive validity of each test.

FCE is thought by many to answer the main concerns of employers: including functional progress of injured workers, and return to work issues, although it sometimes has other uses like pre-employment assessments.

Advantages of FCE

- Identification of abilities helps determine what the patient can achieve
- Provides a comparison between functional capacity and PDC (physical demand classification) levels
- Objectivity – frequently used by claims managers, clinicians and attorneys
- Identifying the point of maximal medical improvement – prevents prolonged, costly, and ineffective rehabilitation

- The employer can work with the injured worker to set goals for return to work. In addition, a guide to the extent that the worker can tolerate the physical demands of his job can be estimated in a report given in the language of the DOT (Dictionary of Occupational Titles, 1991, 4th Edition).

Issue of Reliability

- If we obtain consistent data from FCE studies of our patients – these can be referred to as reliable data.
- But "reliable data" does not necessarily mean that the effort is maximal.
- Thus, consistent data are a necessary but not sufficient condition to determine maximal effort. Inconsistent data, on the other hand, are invariably unreliable.
- We do *not* use FCE to make comments on whether the patient is magnifying the symptoms.
- All we can do is to determine whether the patient's self-reported symptoms are consistent with observed behavior.

Role of FCE in RTW Issues

- Functional testing can reveal the patient's capacities and limitations.
- Functional capacity is compared with norms, and serial assessments are made to monitor progress if necessary.
- Slow or no progress may necessitate more frequent multidisciplinary meetings for evaluation.

Disadvantage of FCE

- It measures *performance not capacity*, and still depends on patient's efforts. Some believe it is much affected by behavior or in essence a behavioral test (particularly when it comes to chronic pain like chronic back pain).
- Expense
- Needs a trained observer
- Time-consuming if a full FCE is performed, may take hours

Recent Doubts Cast on the Usefulness of FCE
(Workers with Chronic LBP)

A recent study found better performance on evaluation was only weakly associated with faster recovery in workers with chronic LBP (Gross and Batt, Spine, 2004). Contrary to functional capacity evaluation theory, better functional capacity evaluation performance, as indicated by a lower number of failed tasks, was in fact associated with higher risk of recurrence. The validity of the FCE's purported ability to identify claimants who are "safe" to return to work is suspect (Gross and Batt, Spine, 2004).

Possible Reason for the Observed Limitations of FCE in LBP

It should be noted that FCEs should be considered behavioral tests influenced by multiple factors, including physical ability, beliefs and perceptions besides the patient's physical status, so FCE does have its limitations (Phys Ther, 2005).

Current Case Scenario

Instead of stressing the use of FCE, you use a more humanitarian approach by the use of COPM (Canadian Ocuupational Performance Measure) and Goal Attaining Scaling as described in the companion text. Your multidisciplinary team works out the immediate, intermediate, and long-term goals for Simpson. At first, we set goals that are easy to attain for the worker as a form of encouragement, at a later stage, more demanding functional tasks and work tasks will be prescribed. Simpson managed to go back to his previous job after 4 months of functional rehabilitation with emphasis on both concentric and eccentric contraction of trunk muscles, and attention to the ergonomics of lifting maneuvers. He was also assessed by the psychiatrist of your multi-disciplinary team, who did not find any significant psychosocial elements contributing to his back pain. It is interesting to note that recent research from UK back pain units also supports the use of the COPM, like the author. This study found that patients with chronic low-back pain report problems with diverse activities. The COPM provides a patient-centered outcome measure that displays good external validity and responsiveness to change when addressing the individual's goals (Spine, 2004).

Learning Point

- Many workers involved in periodic lifting maneuvers, may in fact have the weak "link," located at a time point between concentric and eccentric contraction of the erector spinae muscle of the back or vice versa. In these situations, specific training of both types of contraction as well as ways to effect a more proper and smooth transition between concentric and eccentric activity is required.

- Besides the above, re-training of the frequently weakened local segmental multifidus and transversus abdominis are often needed, as described previously in this book.

- Many workers disabled by chronic LBP need to be assessed by a multidisciplinary team, and the use of the Canadian Occupational Performance Measure and Goal Attainment Scaling often helps in obtaining improvement.

- The term "functional capacity evaluation" (FCE) in popular use often leads different parties involved in a worker's compensation case (e.g., lawyer, case manager, insurance company manager, therapist, patient, and even attorneys) to think that it is a foolproof and objective evaluation of the worker's capacity. In fact, FCE measures performance not capacity, still depends on patient's efforts, and in the case of workers with LBP, Gross reported in Spine 2004 that better functional capacity evaluation performance, as indicated by a lower number of failed tasks, was in fact associated with a higher risk of recurrence of back pain. Thus, FCE is not always a foolproof measure to predict ability to return to work, especially if the hurdle troubling our patient is one of *pain*, since as pointed out earlier, pain behavior often affects the worker's final performance after return to work.

References

1. Gross DP, Batt MC (2004) The prognostic value of functional capacity evaluation in patients with chronic low back pain. II. Sustained recovery. Spine, 29(8):920–924

2. Gross DP, Batt MC (2005) Factors influencing results of functional capacity evaluations in worker's compensation claimants with low back pain. Phys Ther, 85(4):315–322

3. Walsh AD, Kelly JS, et al. (2004) Performance problems of patients with chronic low back pain and the measurement of patient-centered outcome. Spine, 29(1):87–93

Stiffness after Flexor Tendon Repair

History and Examination

You were reviewing more complicated cases presented in a morbidity meeting one day of your department. You came across your junior registrar presenting the case of a 38-year-old laborer Anthony, suffering from a crush injury with open wound of his right ring finger with complete tear of the flexor digitorum profundus at Zone 1 with adequate distal stump and no bony avulsion. The registrar insisted he had tested for the functions of individual flexors of all the fingers, and that he has applied meticulous repair of the FDP and arranged for Anthony to undergo Kleinert's protocol of flexor tendon rehabilitation postoperatively. The presenting problem now at 5 weeks after operation involves right ring finger proximal interphalangeal joint (PIPJ) developing flexion contracture and Anthony also noted some weakness in flexion of the nearby fingers. The junior registrar further commented that the operation was smooth despite the repair being done in the early hours of the morning, although he noted rather high tension and experienced some difficulty in bringing the cut FDP ends together. Describe your comments on this case, with respect to flexor tendon rehabilitation protocol and with respect to the postoperative PIPJ stiffness.

Discussion

Introduction

There is a plethora of postoperative regimens published in the scientific literature on flexor tendon rehabilitation. In a recent article in *Journal of Hand Surgery*, 191 therapists completed a survey. Findings suggested that Kleinert-type and Duran-type regimens are widespread (J Hand Surg, 2005). Hence, these two protocols will be mentioned below. But before review of the protocols, we need to know the mechanics of pertinent basic flexor tendon repair.

Basic Rationale and Concepts in Flexor Tendon Rehabilitation

- Tensile stress on normally repaired flexor tendons is as follows:
  - Passive motion – 500–750 g
  - Light grip – 1,500–2,250 g
  - Strong grip – 5,000–7,500 g
  - Tip pinch, index FDP – 9,000–13,500 g
- Importance of initial period of protection: the strength of the repair is variable over the course of the healing process. Initially rather strong, but the repair strength decreases significantly at days 5–21 after operation.
- Strength of repaired flexors increases rapidly when the repaired tendon is stressed. Controlled stress is applied proportional to increasing tensile strength. Stressed tendons heal faster, gain strength faster, and have fewer adhesions and better excursion. Tensile strength begins to gradually grow stronger at 3 weeks. Generally, blocking exercises are initiated 1 week after active range of motion excursion (at around 5 weeks postoperatively).
- Passive range of motion in extension exercises start 2 weeks after active range of motion excursion (6 weeks postoperatively). Graded excursion strengthening starts 8 weeks postoperatively. If the digital nerve was repaired simultaneously, splint the PIPJ at 30° of flexion in a dorsal-blocking splint. Extension may increase by 10° weekly, starting from the fourth week. No protocol allows forceful use of the hand until the end of the 8th postoperative week. Greatest achievement with range of motion is seen between 12 and 14 weeks after surgery. Unrestricted motion and normal hand use are allowed 12 weeks after the repair.

Kleinert's Rationale

- Kleinert make use of a dorsal-blocking splint (Fig. 37) to place repaired tendons in a protected shortened position to alleviate stress to anastomosis and prevents full active extension. Rubber band traction maintains digits in flexed position. Since rubber bands pull digits back into flexion, this will alleviate any active flexor contraction. Rubber band traction provides tendon excursion to repaired tendons while minimizing stress. Tendon glide during the healing phase minimizes scar adhesions while promoting intrinsic tendon healing. The patient should be observed for fixed flexion contracture of the PIPJ, which sadly happened in this case.

- A well-motivated and reliable patient can initiate a Duran or Indianapolis protocol. Otherwise, Kleinert's protocol is applied, with rubber bands attached to hooks glued to fingernails. However, there is an increasing number of hand surgeons nowadays who refrain from using Kleinert's protocol for digits that have suffered crush injury with lots of edema, the reason being that these digits are very prone to developing PIPJ contracture.

Duran's Protocol

- Duran's protocol is one of the most frequently used and modified by hand therapists in many US centers. If flexion contracture develops, two options exist: initiation of Kleinert's technique or controlled

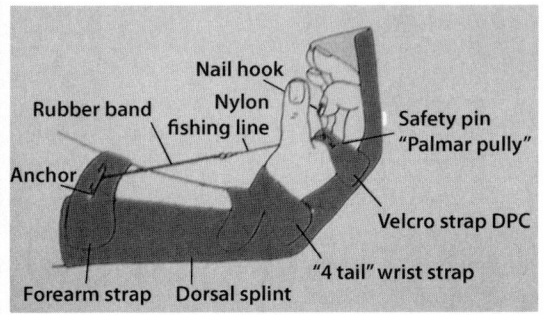

Fig. 37 Design of the Kleinert splint

passive extension of IP joints with the more proximal joints in the protected position of full flexion.

- At surgery, a half (dorsal-blocking) cast is applied with the wrist at 20–30° of flexion, the metacarpal phalangeal (MCP) joints at 70–80° of flexion, and the interphalangeal (IP) joints straight.
- At 1 week, the cast is removed and a dorsal splint is placed. The wrist is held in 20° of flexion, and the MCP joints are held in relaxed flexion. With the MCP and PIP flexed, the distal interphalangeal (DIP) is passively extended. Then, with the DIP and MCP flexed, the PIP is extended.
- After 4–5 weeks, the splint is removed and a wristband with rubber band traction is applied. While awake, the patient passively flexes all joints of the affected finger towards the palm and then actively extends the finger to the splint hood 15–25 times per hour.
- After 5–6 weeks, the patient begins active flexion with wristband removal.
- After 7–8 weeks, the patient begins resisted flexion.

PIP Joint Flexion Contracture

In a recent survey in J Hand Ther 2005, during the rehabilitation of flexor tendon injuries, a PIPJ contracture was reportedly fairly common, but fairly uncommon upon completion of the rehabilitation program. Despite the above, over half of the respondents in this survey who consisted of therapists, reported that their patients had experienced this complication to various extents. Those therapists reporting "never" having encountered the problem of PIPJ contractures in fact turned out to have treated this condition very infrequently.

Present Case Scenario

The phenomenon, as seen in this case, where the FDP was being advanced by more than 1 cm by the junior resident, thus limiting the excursion proximally of the other FDP tendons of the adjacent fingers, is known as the quadrigia effect. Not only can this situation predispose to flexion contracture of the finger thus affected, but can cause decreased flexion power grip of the neighboring digits.

As mentioned, many expert hand surgeons nowadays tend to shy away from the once very popular Kleinert's protocol in the rehabilitation of torn flexor tendons in the face of crush injury in laborers. Since, in these situations, the affected finger tends to become edematous and stiffens quickly, and this tendency is sometimes made worse by an improperly made Kleinert's type of splint.

Stiffness frequently develops under these circumstances at the PIPJ. If we recall the anatomy of the PIPJ, on the volar side, there is the presence of the volar plate with its accompanying thin fiber extensions known by the name of swallow tails. In hands affected by edema, these extensions may become quickly hypertrophied and shortened, as checkrein ligaments. These hypertrophied checkrein ligaments can develop rapidly in the face of edema, particularly with the PIPJ held in flexion.

To tackle the established PIPJ flexion contracture noted during rehabilitation of flexor tendon injuries employing Kleinert's protocol, the

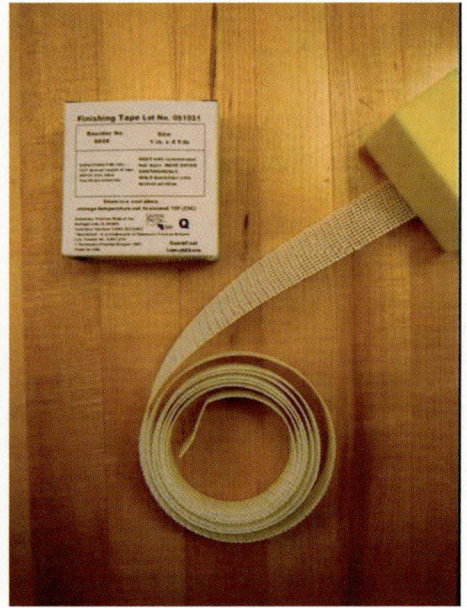

Fig. 38 New material that is quick to apply and provides better comfort used in serial casting as in this case of proximal interphalangeal joint stiffness

author finds the use of serial casting by new light-weight pliable materials useful (Fig. 38).

Learning Point

- The hypertrophied checkrein ligaments of the PIPJ can develop and stiffen rapidly in the face of edema particularly with the PIPJ held in flexion. No matter how well the splint is made in Kleinert's protocol, the PIPJ is still in flexion for the first few weeks, according to the Kleinert's method. This will significantly increase the chance of PIPJ flexion contracture, if, as in this case, the cause of the injury to the flexors is a crushing type of injury.
- Post-repair weakness of adjacent digits on flexion should make one rule out causes like the quadrigia effect, or a missed concomitant injury to the adjacent flexors.
- The current trend is to go for a combination of modified Kleinert's plus modified Duran's protocol. In fact, with proper design of these newer rehabilitation protocols, patient-assisted passive exercises can in fact be very safe and more cost effective than therapist-assisted passive exercises (Am J Phys Med Rehabil, 2001).

References

1. Groth GN (2005) Current practice patterns of flexor tendon rehabilitation. J Hand Ther, 18(2):169–74
2. Cetin A, Cetin M, et al. (2001) Rehabilitation of flexor tendon injuries by use of a combined regimen of modified Kleinert and modified Duran techniques. Am J Phys Med Rehabil, 80(10):721–8

History and Examination

Mrs Jennings came to your office yesterday complaining of persistent back pain after giving birth to her firstborn child 5 months ago. She cannot recall having back troubles in the past, and was perfectly efficient performing her housework, as she stays mostly at home and only her husband works as a pilot. She enjoyed good health in the past apart from an old history of glomerulo-nephritis 15 years ago at a time when she was only 22 years of age. Despite treatment by a local nephrologist, she still has on and off edema of her legs on prolonged walking which has been the main reason for her to stay at home and all along has had little exercise.

On examination, you found that she is healthy looking for a 37-year-old. She does have mild pitting edema of her lower limbs but no sign of cardiovascular or liver disease as the cause of her edema. She has reasonably good flexibility of her lumbar spine in all directions, and no objective lower limb neurological deficit, and there were no sciatic tension signs. However, the bedside Patrick's test was positive on both sides and you found local tenderness posteriorly at both sacroiliac joints, more on the left. Further testing suggested that there is an element of hypermobility of the sacroiliac joint (SIJ) associated with pain. Radiographs were normal, with preserved disc spaces, preserved lordosis and there were no signs of osteitis changes at either SIJ. You performed a diagnostic nerve block to the SIJ, but it turned out to be diagnostic and only partly therapeutic as Mrs Jennings had relapses of her SIJ pain on subsequent clinic follow-ups. You have decided to embark on an exercise program for the patient in view of the partial response of SIJ injections. How would you proceed from here?

Discussion

The sacroiliac joint is an under-appreciated cause of low back and buttock pain. It is thought to cause at least 15% of low back pain. It is more common in the presence of trauma, pregnancy, or in some athletes. The pelvic anatomy is complex, with the joint space being variable and irregular. The joint transmits vertical forces from the spine to the lower extremities and plays a role in lumbo-pelvic dynamic motion. History and physical examination findings can be helpful in screening for sacroiliac joint pain, but individual provocative maneuvers have unproven validity. Fluoroscopically guided injections into the joint have been found to be helpful and SIJ injection is preferred by the author to be very useful because of its diagnostic as well as therapeutic capabilities, sharing the viewpoint with other researchers (Foley and Buschbacher, Am J Phys Med Rehabil, 2006).

Dysfunction in the sacroiliac joint is thought to cause low back and/or leg pain. The pain can be similar to pain caused by a lumbar disc herniation. This condition is generally more common in young and middle-aged women.

While it is not clear how the pain is caused, it is thought that an alteration in the normal joint motion may be the culprit that causes sacroiliac joint pain. This source of pain can be caused by either too little or too much motion.

Pain Generation from the SIJ
- Too much movement – hypermobility or instability, or
- Too little movement – hypomobility or fixation

The pain is typically felt on one side of the low back or buttocks, and can radiate down the leg. The pain usually remains above the knee, but at times pain can extend to the ankle or foot.

Differential Diagnosis

Accurately diagnosing sacroiliac joint dysfunction can be difficult. The symptoms mimic other common conditions, such as disc herniation and radiculopathy.

Possible Pathogenesis of Pregnancy-related SIJ Pain

- Some increase in mobility of the SIJ and the pubic symphysis articulation is noted and may be associated with pelvic pain (Ostgaard, 1997).
- The mechanism is via the release of a high molecular weight hormone, relaxin, coupled with the effects of estrogen (Kristiansson, 1997).
- Consequently, the locking mechanism of the pelvic girdle is less effective, increasing the strain on the ligaments of the SIJ and pubic symphysis.
- Normally, the pelvic girdle takes between 3 and 6 months post-delivery to return to the pre-pregnant state.
- There are reports that some ladies have persistent pelvic pain beyond this period (Heiberg and Aarseth, 1997), such as this patient – initiation of an appropriate exercise program is recommended.

Common Treatment Options

Typical treatments for sacroiliac joint dysfunction include:

- Sacroiliac joint injections (Fig. 39)
- Physical therapy and exercise (see below)
- Hydrotherapy

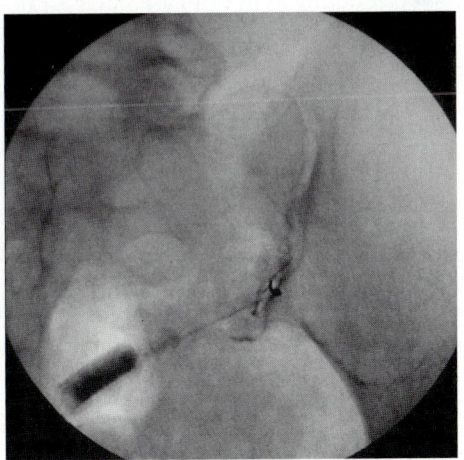

Fig. 39 Radiograph showing fluoroscopic-guided sacro-iliac joint injection for this patient

Rationale and Administration of Exercise Therapy

- Pregnancy-related ligament laxity does take time to recover.
- The transversus got stretched during the 9 months since conception and needs to be retrained.
- Hyperlordosis, if present, may exacerbate shear forces on L5/S1 and worsen any pre-existing pathologies there.
- Dynamic stabilizer training of the SIJ, besides re-training of the transversus and multifidus as well as pelvic floor plus diaphragm is important here:
  - Posteriorly: Strengthens the ipsilateral gluteus maximus plus contralateral latissimus dorsi (this helps decrease hypermobility via the intervening thoraco-dorsal fascia, according to anatomic studies by Vleeming)
  - Anteriorly: Strengthens the ipsilateral hip adductors plus contralateral internal oblique and external oblique via the intervening anterior abdominal fascia
  - Laterally: Strengthens the ipsilateral hip adductors plus the contralateral gluteus medius and minimus muscles

Overall Role of SIJ Injections

- SIJ injections can be both diagnostic and therapeutic.
- If the cause of pain is from hypermobility as in this case, then SIJ injection is done only if the diagnosis is unsure. The mainstay of management is by exercise therapy as mentioned. SIJ injections are found by the author to be more useful in cases of hypomobility and in such cases can indeed serve the function of helping to clinch the diagnosis as well as having a therapeutic effect.

Current Case Scenario

Mrs Jennings had marked improvement after the combined use of sacroiliac joint injections and exercise therapy. You referred her for hydrotherapy after completion of exercise therapy and when she was pain-free.

Learning Point

- The sacroiliac joint is a well-innervated diarthrodial synovial joint with the capability of being a source of low back pain and referred pain in the lower extremity. There are no definite historical, physical, or radiological features to provide a definite, foolproof diagnosis of sacroiliac joint pain, although many authors have advocated provocational maneuvers to suggest the SIJ as a pain generator, such as the Patrick's test. An accurate diagnosis is made by controlled SIJ diagnostic blocks and is favored by the author; this view is also shared by others.

- Programmed rehabilitation by the exercise therapy described is of benefit, especially to those scenarios of pregnancy-related SIJ hypermobility as the cause of pain.

References

1. Hansen HC, McKenzie-Brown AM (2007) Sacroiliac joint interventions: a systematic review. Pain Physician, 10(1):165–84
2. Foley BS, Buschbacher RM (2006) Sacroiliac joint pain: biomechanics, diagnosis, and treatment. Am J Phys Med Rehabil, 85(12):997–1006
3. Mooney V, Vleeming A (2007) Movement, stability, and lumbopelvic pain: Integration of research and therapy. 2nd edition, Churchill Livingstone

History and Examination

Johnson is a 28-year-old company executive in a local bank, his father being the CEO of the same bank. Johnson is active in sports including bicycling, driving, and sailing. He is a member of the international bicycling team representing his country. Four months ago, Johnson was driving his new Lotus sports car on the motorway when it ran into a truck. Johnson found his left leg got trapped in the car wreckage and could not move. He was rushed to the nearest general hospital where emergency transfemoral amputation was performed as his left lower extremity from the knee downward was beyond salvage. Postoperatively, Johnson was nursed in the ICU for treatment of acute renal failure secondary to crush syndrome and myoglobinuria. Johnson subsequently made a full recovery and he was transferred to your rehabilitation unit. There was phantom sensation, but no pain, the transfemoral amputation stump was well, and there was no flexion or adduction contracture. Johnson received physical and occupational therapy. You initially trained him on a simple single-axis prosthesis followed by arrangement by the high end advanced knee prosthesis marketed as Rheo Knee by the company Ossur using breakthrough microprocessor technology and partly designed by MIT with the use of magneto-rheological fluid. This prosthesis was chosen because Johnson managed very well with the use of a traditional, single-axis knee prosthesis, he belonged to high level K4 functional classification, and is determined to lead a more active lifestyle despite his amputation.

Discussion

Introduction

The functional K-classification system originating from the United States Health Care Financing Administration (HCFA) common procedure coding system gives a good description of the functional disabilities of amputees. Patients with a high functional K-classification level may benefit from new advanced prosthetic knee technologies made possible via the use of microprocessor technology such as the Otto-bock C-leg and Ossur's Rheo Knee. In these advanced knee systems, there is continuous adjustment of swing resistance up to 50 times each second.

Although these advanced systems have both pneumatic and hydraulic systems available, the hydraulic system is used more often. Advanced knee systems help high functional level amputees to negotiate stairs, recovery from stumbling, prevent falls, make stance flexion possible with thus better shock absorption, and are cadence responsive, thus reducing conscious effort and stress for the user to maintain knee stability during gait.

Ossur's Rheo Knee

This prosthetic knee system (Fig. 40) samples loading and joint position of the knee at a rate of 1,000 times per second during stance then adjusts resistance accordingly. Stance flexion and extension resistance are adjusted by the microprocessor based on joint position, load, and velocity. Rheo Knee automatically identifies slow, moderate, and fast walking speeds and updates flexion and extension resistance values. The HP iPAQ personal digital assistant in conjunction with Rheo Logic software allows for programming of the Rheo Knee and monitoring of system utilities. When making adjustments with the PDA, one should make sure that the user is seated or in a stable standing position. All Rheo Knee functions, including stance phase stability, are interrupted during the period in which the settings are updating and data are being transferred from the PDA to the Rheo Knee. Recommended dynamic response feet that are compatible with the Rheo Knee system include the Ceterus, Vari-Flex, Talux, and Elation.

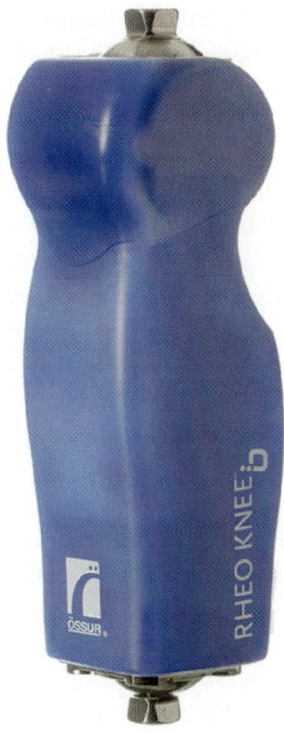

Fig. 40 The actual Rheo Knee prosthesis (picture courtesy of Ossur)

Five Levels of the Functional Classification System

- K0 = unable to ambulate or transfer safely with or without assistance; a prosthesis does not enhance quality of life or mobility
- K1 = mainly household ambulator, may use a prosthesis for transfer or ambulation on level surfaces at a fixed cadence
- K2 = limited community ambulator, may be capable of using the prosthesis to negotiate low-level environmental barriers, e.g., curb, stairs, uneven surfaces
- K3 = community ambulator, with potential to achieve ambulation with variable cadence, negotiate most environmental barriers; may achieve prosthetic use beyond simple locomotion

- K4 = typical of prosthetic demands of the child, athlete, or very active adult. Having the potential to exceed basic ambulation skills, and participate in activities of high impact, stress and energy levels

Use of "Smart Material" in Ossur's Rheo Knee

Smart materials have one or more properties that can be dramatically altered. Most everyday materials have physical properties, which cannot be significantly altered; whereas a smart material with variable viscosity may turn from a fluid that flows easily into a solid. A variety of smart materials already exist, and are being researched extensively. These include piezo-electric materials, magneto-rheostatic materials, electro-rheostatic materials, and shape memory alloys. Each individual type of smart material has a different property that can be significantly altered, such as viscosity, volume, and conductivity. The property that can be altered influences what types of applications the smart material can be used for. Magneto rheostatic fluids are being developed for use in car shocks, damping washing machine vibration, prosthetic limbs, exercise equipment, and surface polishing of machine parts. This type of magneto-rheostatic fluid is used in the Rheo Knee system and provides frictional resistance to flexion and extension movement. Advantages include very low torque production during the swing phase, allows for easy initiation of knee flexion, zero pressure actuator has the potential for a long lifetime of use and low maintenance requirements, actuator weight is located more proximal in the knee, providing a light-weight feel during the swing phase. For readers interested in the rheological properties of magneto-rheological fluids the article by Park et al. is recommended (J Colloid Interface Sci, 2001).

Current Case Scenario

Prior to the decision to arrange the Ossur's Rheo Knee system for Johnson, you ensured that Johnson has adequate knee stability in controlling a single-axis prosthetic knee through voluntary control and active hip extension. This good degree of voluntary control is needed not only when the Rheo Knee is powered off, but also during its functional use as the alignment reference line of the Rheo Knee is positioned more posterior to the knee center; the user will experience more stance flexion during the loading response and good muscular control of the amputee is an absolute prerequisite before the Rheo Knee can be used to its full potential. Last, but not the least important, you referred Johnson to participate in the mutual-sharing gait training and certification courses run by the company Ossur to further increase your patient's confidence in the use of his high-technology knee prosthesis.

Learning Point

- Electro-rheostatic (ER) and magneto-rheostatic (MR) materials are fluids that can experience a dramatic change in their viscosity. These fluids can change from a thick fluid to nearly a solid substance within the span of a millisecond when exposed to a magnetic or electric field; the effect can be completely reversed just as quickly when the field is removed. MR fluids experience a viscosity change when exposed to a magnetic field, while ER fluids experience similar changes in an electric field. The most common form of magneto-rheostatic fluid consists of tiny iron particles suspended in oil.

- Magneto-rheological fluids such as these are also used in other applications, such as in a force feedback glove reported by Bouzit for use in haptic and force feedback in virtual reality platforms, which is to be discussed briefly in the next section.

- Smart materials also find applications in the prosthetics industry, such as the development of novel materials (electroactive polymers) that are not only light-weight and quiet, but potentially act as both sensors and actuators at the same time. One such material is the dielectric elastomer artificial muscle. If successful, the use of these electroactive polymers can potentially offer a light-weight, pliable, yet soundless alternative to current prosthetics, which are bulky, heavy, with sound-producing cams and gears.

References

1. Park JH, Chin BD, et al. (2001) Rheological properties and stabilization of magneto-rheological fluids in a water-in-oil emulsion. J Colloid Interface Sci, 240(1):349–354
2. Winter SH, Bouzit M (2007) Use of magnetorheologic fluid in a force feedback glove. IEEE Trans Neural Syst Rehabil Eng, 15:1, 2–8

Use of Virtual Environments in Orthopedic Rehabilitation

General Introduction

Once upon a time, a little child asked his teacher after a physics lesson the question: "Why do we think our world is real?" The teacher answered: "Of course our world is real, can you not feel your textbook and the pile of homework that I gave you, did you not see the beauty of the setting sun last evening, or can you not hear the singing of birds now that I am walking you through the park, filled with the smell of roses?"

The child happens to be the author when he was young. What the teacher says is in fact quite true to the great majority of us: We think we are in a real physical world because we can interact, and get feedback from the physical world that we live in. Similarly, in the computer-simulated virtual world that is often referred to as "virtual reality," the more friendly the environment created by the computer and the more sensory feedback one gets, i.e., visual, touch, sound, even smell, etc., the higher the chance the person will think he is in fact part of the virtual world. The execution is not easy, but this should be the aim of any virtual reality (VR) system especially those that are put to medical use like the training of surgeons, or rehabilitation of patients.

As far as VR is concerned, experts like Burdea have taught us that there are three key cornerstones: Immersion, Interaction, and Imagination (Burdea et al., IEEE Trans Rehabil Eng, 2000). This is easy to explain: To be successful, the user should be absorbed into the virtual world, thinking he is part of it, i.e., Immersion; this Immersion comes about by being able to Interact with the virtual word, especially visual real-time changes of graphics and provision of touch (haptic) and force feedbacks; the rest will be Imagination, which is helped by the use of high-end scene graphs and toolkits designed for virtual reality platforms. Before we talk about VR, we need to briefly review the uses of the computer in orthopedics in a more general sense.

Uses of the Computer in Orthopedics

Some of the important uses of the computer were mentioned in different companion texts by the same author. In the book *Orthopedic Traumatology – a Resident's Guide*, the author talks about the use of CT-based navigation and especially the use of virtual fluoroscopy. In the latter technique, a virtual model of the skeletal part is stored in the computer so that the amount of radiation to which the surgeon is subjected will be decreased; by the same token, saving the virtual skeletal part in many different planes can aid intraoperative guidance of the performance and placement of strategic screws in difficult areas, such as sacro-iliac screws in SIJ disruptions (Fig. 41) in the case of fractured pelvis and anterior column acetabular screws in cases of acetabular fractures (Fig. 42).

Obviously the use of the computer and associated software has benefited the orthopedic surgeons in other aspects, such as preoperative planning (will be discussed), preoperative 3D imaging (Fig. 43), intraoperative computer navigation in total joint and spine surgery, besides trauma surgery as mentioned above, more recently, virtual intraoperative impingement and stability testing in ACL reconstruction in the field of sports medicine. Also, elaborate computer systems are now available in well-developed nations like the UK and USA to help prevent musculoskeletal disorders arising from the prolonged use of visual-display

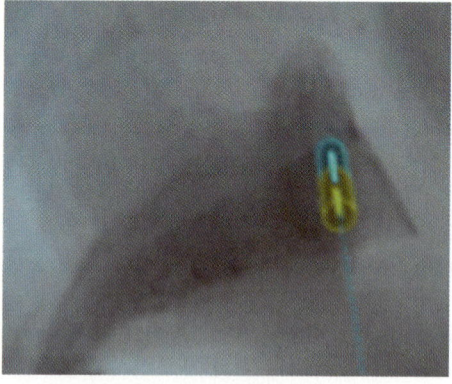

Fig. 41 Virtual fluoroscopic-aided insertion of sacro-iliac screws

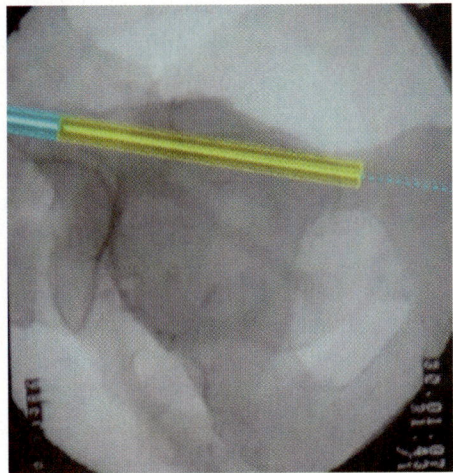

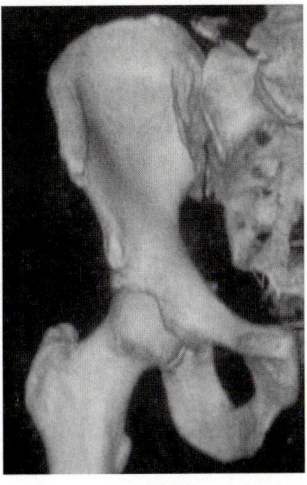

Fig. 42 Virtual fluoroscopic-aided insertion of screw at the anterior column of the acetabulum

Fig. 43 Use of three-dimensional CT software gives us a better visual of fractures in more challenging areas like the pelvis, as in this case

units such as computer workstations via an on-line system consisting of e-learning, occupational health and risk assessments, e-mail reminders, and periodic health monitoring of workers, and channeling abnormal results to on-site health workers for follow-up actions. Before ending this section, let us not forget the growing importance and emerging tendency to store three-dimensional images in our databases for the future of patients who have gone through very complex and difficult reconstruction procedures. There is a good saying that a picture is worth thousands of words. As far as an operative record of complex reconstruction cases is concerned, keeping a 3D instead of a 2D intra-operative digital image goes a long way in helping subsequent surgeons managing the patient if future reconstruction is needed, and is far superior than just relying on three or four descriptive paragraphs of a standard operative record typed by surgeons or their secretaries. Similarly, resected surgical specimens, including tumor specimens, can be quickly scanned into a 3D model with the advent of current technology and the use of high-end 3D laser scanners with dual cameras for proper filing to be used later in conferences, teaching sessions, planning of future reconstructions, and so forth.

Emerging Importance of Data Storage and Retrieval

Computed tomography, or CT, greatly facilitates 3D viewing of the internal morphology of soft tissue and skeletal structures. Units will soon begin to appear in dental offices for use in oral surgery, orthodontics, and implants.

The same can apply to storing important information for our orthopedic patients, such as storing in 3D relevant intraoperative features, such as status of soft tissue and bony elements after tumor resection. This will facilitate subsequent re revisions of skeletal/soft tissue reconstruction, or tumor reconstruction. Properly filing the intraoperative data as well as having a 3D model of resected, say, tumor specimens, will also be valuable if the case turns into a medico-legal matter afterwards.

The new technologies that allow quick transformation of a 3D object to be scanned into the computer so that we can view the 3D object later on any time we like will be discussed shortly, together with the advent of new 3D scanners.

Why Develop Virtual Reality?

In the author's opinion, VR can tackle three main difficult areas in clinical medicine:

- Avoiding unnecessary risk to patients by practicing surgical skills on virtual patients, while at the same time improving the techniques of trainee surgeons, and avoiding radiation risks to orthopedic surgeons in the case of virtual fluoroscopy.
- From the point of view of orthopedic rehabilitation, VR helps overcome practical hurdles of some patients who are not participating in rehabilitation because of long distances involved in traveling to hos-

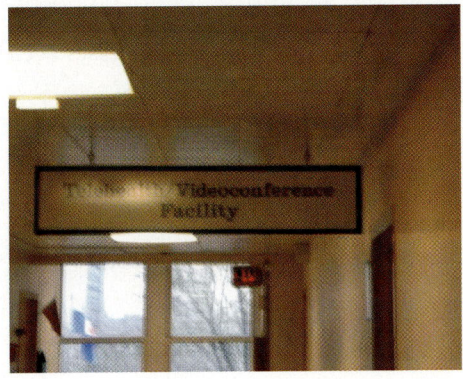

Fig. 44 Tele-health centers are increasing in popularity: pictured is the Telehealth and Video-conferencing facility of the Hospital for Sick Children in Canada

pitals besides cost concerns in so doing, and compliments nicely the already established tele-health centers of major hospitals (Fig. 44), as well as a small but significant group of patients who have "no spare time" for attending therapy sessions, in which case home-based rehabilitation can still proceed as long as there is a telephone line and the right computer system in some cases as illustrated in the various case scenarios in this section.

- Aiding psychosocial rehabilitation in the future in the rehabilitation of many chronic disabilities. Examples include chronic pain patients with social withdrawal and social isolation (training of social interaction and behavior has already been started by some researchers in this field), burn care, especially in young patients who cannot tolerate the pain of treatment (physiotherapy and wound care) besides the danger of social isolation and withdrawal due to, say, facial burns and accompanying disfigurement, etc. These and other examples will be discussed separately as case examples. But first, let us recapitulate a little about the computer technique of VR itself.

Summarizing the Four Main Advantages of Virtual Reality

- Many patients with disabilities appear capable of motor learning within virtual environments.

- Movements learned by people with disabilities in VR transfer to real-world equivalent motor tasks in most cases, and in some cases even generalize to other untrained tasks.
- In the few studies in the literature that have compared motor learning in real versus virtual environments, some advantage of VR training has been found in all cases.
- No occurrences of cyber-sickness in impaired populations have been reported to date in experiments where VR has been used to train motor abilities.

Key Components of a Virtual Reality Platform

This includes the VR engine hardware, accompanying software and databases, input and output devices, user's interface, and one or more designated tasks in mind in the setting of rehabilitative training.

Evolution

In the past, limitations of picture display systems using shutter glasses and primitive software have created image lag due to inadequate computer power, particularly the cheaper systems that strained the users' eyes and made them suffer from dizziness. Since that time, there have been significant advances and cost-reducing developments in both image projection systems and computer performance. These, coupled with large strides made in computer engineering in all aspects, permit the smooth execution and running of the virtual environment.

Forms of Virtual Reality

The term "pure" virtual reality refers to an enveloping artificially constructed world composed solely of computer-created elements with the exception of the people involved. In pure VR, the surface appearance of the person engaged may even be transformed by design. In this form of VR, the person engaged interacts solely with the computer, and not with other human beings or real objects.

Modifications to Suit Training in Surgery and Rehabilitation: Concept of Mixed or Augmented Reality

Mixed virtual reality, sometimes abbreviated as "mixed reality" or called "augmented reality," is either a real-world setting with sizable superimposed and engaging virtual objects, or a computer-simulated setting with sizable superimposed and engaging real components beyond just those participating. Putting it another way, augmented reality is a particular type of VR system where synthetic graphics, images or text, are being registered and overlaid onto the real scene usually using a special device called the see-through head mount display, or cameras and graphics composition systems. Mixed reality environments may have only a few virtual objects, but these components should appear real and cognitively significant for one participant.

Many of the following illustrative case scenarios involve mixed reality since this form of mixed or augmented reality is the form of VR commonly used in patient rehabilitation, which forms the main theme of this book.

Uses of Virtual Reality in Orthopedic Surgery and Rehabilitation

The three main potential uses of virtual reality in medicine have just been discussed. But one should realize that many important databases stem from projects like "The Visible Human Project" (Fig. 45), which was established by the National Library of Medicine to create anatomically detailed, three-dimensional representations of the human body. In the current phase transverse CT, MRI and cryo-sectional images at 1-mm intervals are available. Based on these, one can segment and

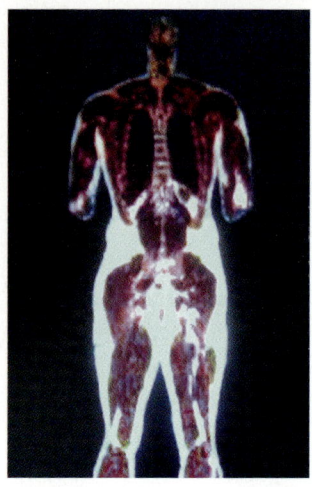

Fig. 45 Computer-aided generation of images from visible human projects that can be viewed in quick time from the net

visualize parts of the human body using digital image processing and computer graphics. All these important projects are dedicated to the improvement of medical education.

Advances in Hardware

The hardware is often the key to the set-up of a virtual reality platform, as it reads and assesses the inputs, gets access to the task-oriented databases, provides feedback and effects constant updating and re-computing the virtual world around every 30 ms (Fig. 46). Latency should be as short as possible to prevent deterioration of simulation quality, and providing real-time updates.

Real-time means the computer is able to detect the user's input and modify the virtual world instantaneously. (The refresh rate must be high or else there will be no feeling of immersion on the part of the subject. To increase the sense of reality, feedback from the virtual environment is important, such as the use of force feedback gloves, as we shall see). Most important determining factors of real-time update include the speed of the CPU and built-in graphic card rendering capability.

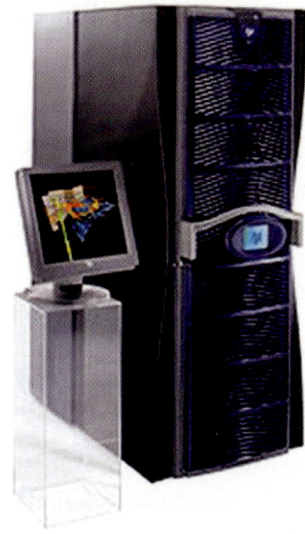

Fig. 46 High-end computer hardware and rendering systems from silicon graphics (courtesy of Silicon Graphics)

The above reinforces the important concept that through the process of "interaction" that enhanced degree of "immersion" will occur.

The hardware, during execution of its function, also needs to convert 3D geometrical models to 2D scenes to effect real-time rendering. The main frame does not only need to effect a graphics-rendering pipeline, but other modalities like a haptics-rendering pipeline.

Advances in Software

As mentioned, optimizing the simulation software will also go a long way in effecting real-time rendering as discussed, and help in the smoothness of execution and prevention of bottlenecks.

To this end, the use of high-end PC graphics accelerators such as the popular NVIDIA Quadro2 Pro or Wildcat II 5110 will be an advantage.

Another important indispensable piece of software is the use of toolkits and scene graphs to create the run-time environment for subsequent real-time interaction by the subject in the virtual world.

Probably the two most popular toolkits are the WorldToolKit and Java 3D. The former is versatile since it supports many commercial I/O (input-output) devices. Java 3D, developed by Sun Microsystems, is also popular and is used in high-end virtual reality research laboratories such as the DISCOVER lab (distributed and collaborative virtual environments research laboratory) at the University of Ottawa.

The Process of Pipeline Synchronization

The process of synchronization is important since it tries to smoothly combine different types of sensorial feedbacks in the virtual simulation to ensure the user's immersion into the virtual environment.

Pipeline synchronization is therefore important to ensure smooth real-time execution of virtual environments. One may use additional CPUs to accomplish the above, or multi-pipeline graphic cards like the Wildcat II 5110 board.

Advances in Input-output Devices

Improving Visual Effects and Depth Perception

Computer graphics in a virtual reality platform are usually projected as a floating image around 3–15 feet (0.9 to 4.5 m) in front of the user wearing the head mount (Fig. 47). Displays can thus be designed for single or multiple users of large-volume displays. Display can also be projected for both eyes or to a single eye (if the patient has impairment in one eye). Nowadays, most VR stations use high-resolution stereoscopic HMD (head mount displays). Techniques to enhance perception of depth are beyond the scope of this book. Discussion of techniques to enhance depth perception is outside the scope of the book, but essentially is based on the use of stereo and binocular disparity of projection of images to the retina of both eyes, and the use of screen parallax. Take the case of HMD, for example. HMD usually employs two separate display devices providing isolated displays for each eye. Two separate im-

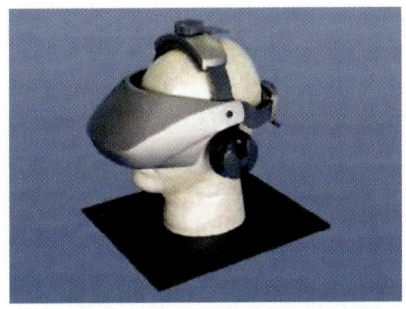

Fig. 47 Illustration showing state-of-the-art HMD 800 series from fifth dimension technologies (Courtesy of 5DT.com)

ages are fed into the respective display channel to create the stereo effect, and increase the feeling of reality and hence immersion.

Quick Scanning of 3D Objects
Subsequently Used in the Virtual World

One of the high-end products with the capability of quickly scanning a 3D object to the computer has been developed by Polhemus.com and is called FastSCAN (Fig. 48). FastSCAN can instantly acquire 3D surface images when you sweep the handheld laser scanning wand over an object, in a manner similar to spray painting. FastSCAN works by

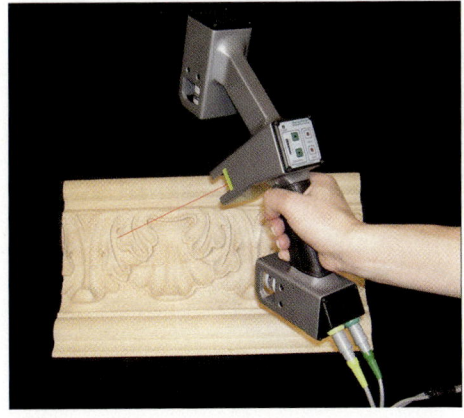

Fig. 48 An example of a 3D scanner marketed by Polhemus.com

projecting a fan of laser light on the object while the camera views the laser to record cross-sectional depth profiles. The object's image immediately appears on your computer screen. Because FastSCAN provides real-time visual feedback, monitoring and controlling the scan process are straightforward. Unlike other scanners, FastSCAN automatically stitches your scans together, saving a great deal of time. The sweeps list enables turning individual sweeps on and off to facilitate optimizing the amount of data in your final output.

Other discussion on geometric and physical modeling and the way to execute depth perception inside a virtual environment is outside the scope of this book, as mentioned.

Virtual 3D Sound Effects Vs. Stereo Sound Effects

Some experts are of the opinion that "creating a realistic sound setting for VR is usually easier than creating realistic 3D pictures or realistic tactile and motion interface. A good surround-sound audio system with several speakers can give high performance surround-sounds to accompany parts and events in virtual reality."

However, very high-end VR sound displays should have the effect on the user that the sound is really emitting from a particular virtual object. More primitive VR stations may still use a 3D sound card, but the current 3D sound technology is based on the difference in energy distribution in the frequency domain of the sound waves, which has led to the development of HRTF (head-related transfer function) technology, which produces spatial sound with energy distributions according to the location of the sound sources for the right and the left ear. Accuracy of the reproduction of 3D sound also requires the location of the user to be tracked and input relayed to the sound synthesis system. The latest state-of-the-art devices will include devices like HURON 3D audio stations.

Importance of the Use of Haptic and Force Feedbacks in Orthopedic Rehabilitation

When simulating the characteristics of touch and motion, VR platforms must simulate the resistance that virtual things would have on

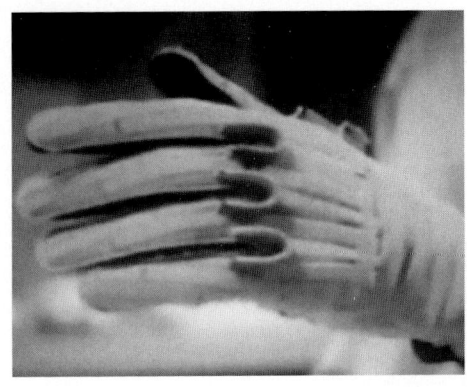

Fig. 49 Tiny micro-pressure sensors can be incorporated into cyber gloves such as the one illustrated, as marketed by immersion.com

motion by body parts such as fingers, arms, and legs. For instance, if one lifts a virtual ball, then one's hand and arm must feel the appropriate resistance as needed in order for the virtual ball to seem real. Pressure sensation can be transmitted from a computer to one's body though micro-pressure sensors (tiny pistons, inflatable bubbles, etc.) powered by mechanical motors, magnetism, hydraulics, or other media. These micro-pressure machines can be integrated into gloves (Fig. 49) or body suits. Direct resistance from 3D fields may be achieved in the coming years. Touch and motion-based computer-to-human communication will become widespread with scientific advances, but it currently lags behind interaction through sight and hearing, or in other words visual and audio-feedbacks. However, one high-end commercial firm specializing in touch-related (haptic) technologies is immersion.com.

Haptic Vs. Force Feedbacks

It should be noted that "haptic (touch) feedback" is not the same as "force feedback." Contrary to force feedback, haptic feedback only conveys real-time information on the surface roughness, temperature, and geometry of objects. Force feedbacks give the user an idea of the object inertia, weight, resistance, etc. In other words, a force feedback interface interacts with the muscles and tendons to give the user of VR a sensation that a force is being applied.

In the field of orthopedic rehabilitation, many virtual reality platforms use force feedbacks such as the robotic arm shown in Fig. 50 developed by MIT (Massachusetts Institute of Technology), and the CyberGrasp force feedback glove by immersion.com (Fig. 51).

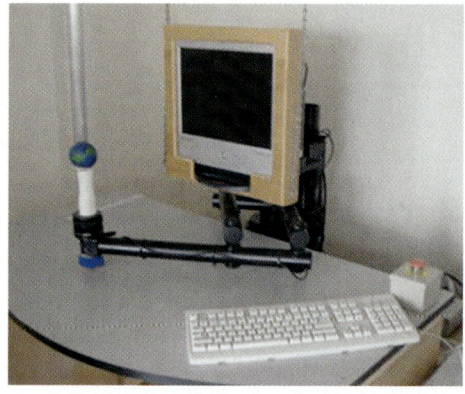

Fig. 50 Example of a robotic arm developed by MIT

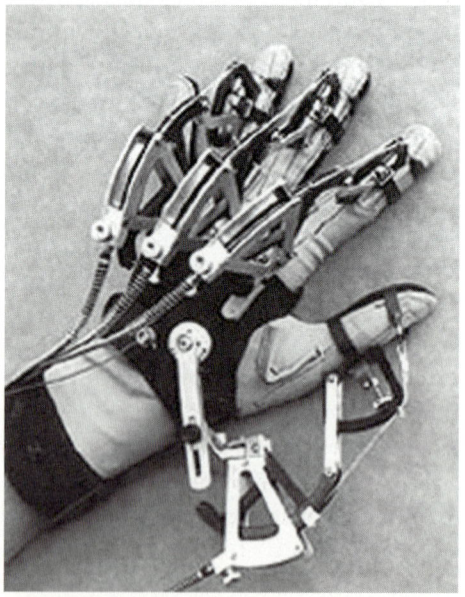

Fig. 51 The state-of-the-art CyberGrasp force feedback glove developed by the pioneering company immersion.com

Interface of Interaction

In the case of the hand for example, this is by means of gestures. For instance, fiber-optic sensors allow the computer to measure thumb and finger bending; thus, interaction is possible through different hand gestures on the part of the user.

Early models of these sensing gloves lacked haptic and force feedbacks, but newer models on the market, such as those sold by immersion.com, are equipped with these.

Other Modalities Besides Vision, Hearing, and Force Feedbacks

These may include other senses such as smell and taste, but will not be discussed in this book.

Way Finding in Virtual Environments

- Virtual interface technology makes it possible to explore spaces without actually being in them.
- The consequent investigation into the study of virtual way finding has emerged from the technological advances of the past decade, and is deemed essential knowledge in the virtual training of surgical techniques in future generations of surgeons. While we will not go too deeply into the technical aspects, we need at least to note the role and users of trackers.

Different Types of Trackers

Trackers are important for they allow detection of real-time change in 3D position of an object in question. They come in many different types:

- Optical: Active vs. passive
- Magnetic
- Ultrasound
- Others: e.g., mechanical/inertial/hybrids that involve at least two motion tracking technologies

Reality inside virtual environments can be enhanced if there is an enhanced tracker update rate, and hence latency for detection should be short. Thus, optical ones have shorter latency than ultrasound ones since the speed of light travels faster than sound waves, while magnetic trackers are subject to interference from nearby electro-magnetic devices.

Passive optical trackers are usually used in some primitive motion analysis system like that used in gait analysis (Fig. 52). Active systems work by LED (light emitting diodes; Fig. 53).

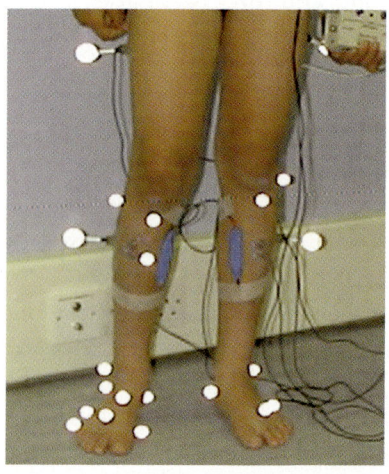

Fig. 52 Picture showing an example of "passive" optical trackers as used in many gait analysis systems

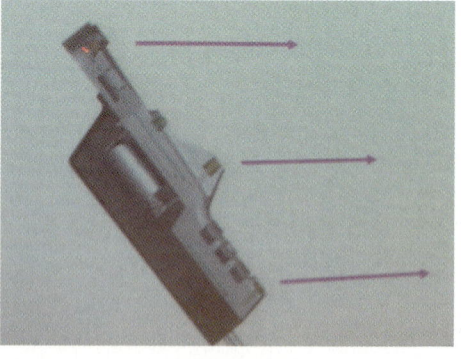

Fig. 53 Picture showing an "active" optical tracker system in the form of light emitting diodes, here marketed by stryker.com

In VR platforms, trackers serve more functions than simply detecting the user's head or hand, etc., instead they often become a navigation interface. Examples include 3D mouse, 3D probes, trackballs, etc.

More elaborate gesture interfaces will be discussed in the setting of the virtual hand. An example is the state-of-the-art CyberGlove by immersion.com, which can be equipped with haptic feedback to the patient.

Preoperative Training of Surgeons

In the future, there will be a tendency toward the training of medical students via the use of a virtual model of the human anatomy, including male and females. Thanks to the collaborative effects of the University of Colorado and National Library of Medicine, a male and female cadaver were imaged by CT and MRI, frozen, sliced and imaged, as mentioned in the "Visible Human Project." Subsequent researchers like Lorensen from General Electric then made use of the visible human volumetric datasets to extract 3D shapes and animations. Students of medicine can learn through these and other 3D animations of virtual anatomy. An example of such virtual anatomy courses is taught at the University of California at San Diego. After students graduate and become trainee surgeons, there are procedures that may be risky when performed for the first few times on patients. An example is the performance of tracheotomy in general surgery. Thus, virtual training of trainee surgeons before such procedures via a virtual reality platform is available in Canada (Fig. 54). Similarly, even larger scale training of general surgeons via virtual reality platforms involving 10,000 trainees has taken place in big organizations like the European Surgical Institute in Germany.

Preoperative Planning

A preoperative model is essential in many challenging, complex reconstructions, or may potentially increase the accuracy of performance of procedures that require quite a high degree of accuracy. An example is

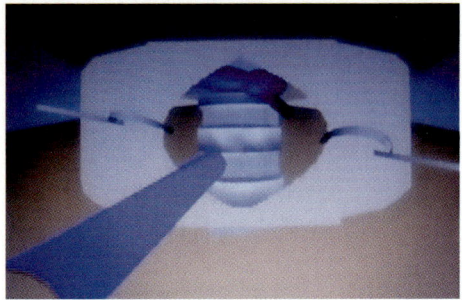

Fig. 54 Use of virtual reality for trainee surgeons in the performance of a procedure with a risk like tracheotomy

the use of preoperative virtual cuts in cases of presurgical planning of high tibial osteotomy (Fig. 55). Similarly, preoperative planning of the best virtual positioning in attempted hip resurfacing (Fig. 56) as far as placement of a prosthesis in pre-existing hip dysplasia-related OA in the hips of young adults is currently being practiced in some units in Japan.

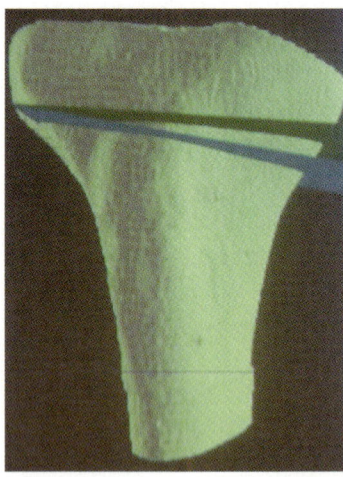

Fig. 55 Performance of a virtual osteotomy on the computer-generated proximal tibia before the real performance of high tibial osteotomy

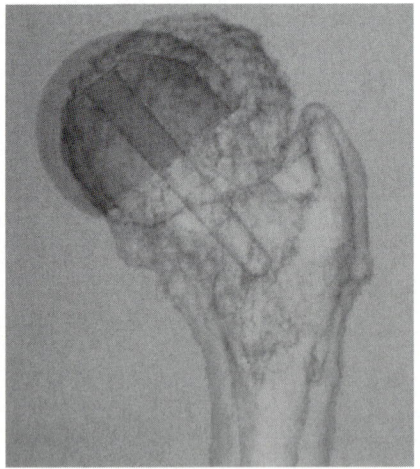

Fig. 56 Preoperative planning of the placement of hip resurfacing prosthesis upon the computer-generated proximal femur of the patient (courtesy of Dr. J. Higashi)

Intraoperative Virtual Model

Building an intraoperative virtual model of the local skeleton, especially of body regions with more complex anatomy such as the pelvis and acetabular areas, or placement of pedicle screws (Fig. 57) where standard landmarks become blurred from previous posterior surgery, is an especially useful guide for the surgeon. The use of virtual fluoroscopy can help make the surgeon put the necessary screws in the right direction and position in areas with a low margin of errors, yet with much less radiation expected from standard continuous fluoroscopic screening.

Intra- or Perioperative Stability/Impingement Testing in Other Fields of Orthopedic Surgery

Real-time impingement control and stability testing can be useful in peri- and intraoperative testing during ACL reconstruction and managing more challenging cases of THR. Take ACL reconstruction as an example, virtual fluoroscopy can effect fluoro-based femoral and tibial tunnel planning (Fig. 58). For single tunnel reconstruction, the quadrant method by Bernard Hertel can be used, while in cases of double bundle, the method by Imhoff/Lorenz of using a planning grid can be considered. Virtual fluoroscopy can also perform fluoro-based pre-drill-

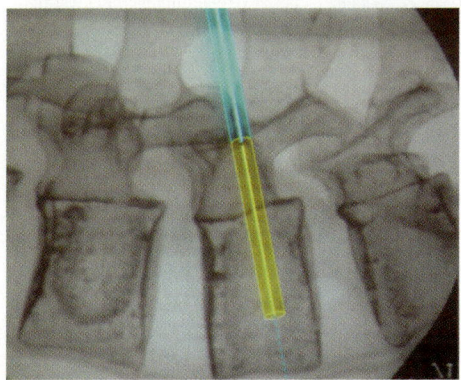

Fig. 57 Placement of pedicle screw trajectory on intraoperative virtual model of the vertebral column of the patient, developed by stryker.com

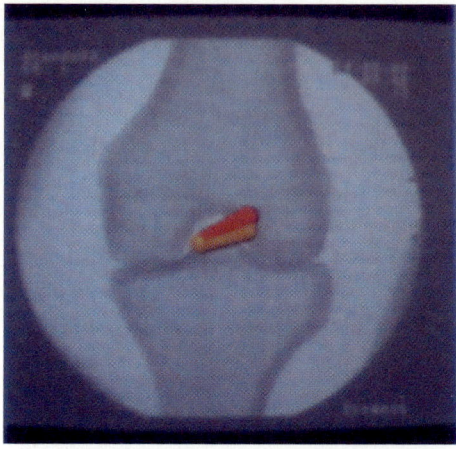

Fig. 58 Virtual fluoroscopic-based intraoperative checks of anterior cruciate ligament tunnel positioning

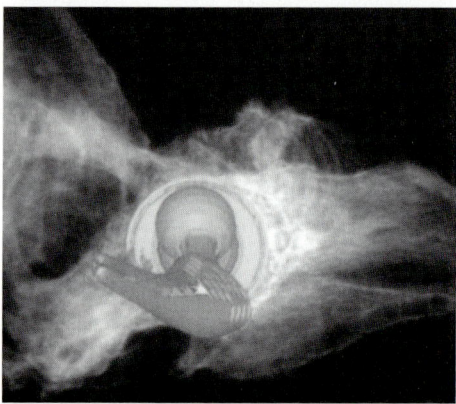

Fig. 59 Subtle instability from impingement revealed by this CT-based virtual impingement testing (courtesy of Dr. J. Higashi)

ing and perform virtual impingement testing. Software with built-in impingement warnings can exercise fluoro-based image free pre- and post-reconstruction stability testing. On the other hand, CT-based virtual impingement testing can be useful during, say, revision of THR for previous recurrent dislocation in which the cause was suspected to be one of impingement, and subtle impingement/stability issues may be revealed in various joint positions (Fig. 59).

An Intraoperative Aid to the Surgeon Combined with Robotics

Medical robotics in combination with VR interfaces enables surgery on a micro-scale with more precision than traditional operating procedures, as well as on a macro-scale in other situations.

In the field of total joint surgery, peri- or intraoperative virtual drilling of the proposed track of the intramedullary canal by a medical robot can be considered in more difficult and challenging scenarios such as altered proximal canal anatomy of the proximal femur. Figure 60 shows the pre-planned proposed track of reaming by the use of an intraoperative robotic arm.

Use of Virtual Reality in Postoperative Orthopedic Rehabilitation

The following is an example of postoperative rehabilitation aided by virtual reality in the field of hand rehabilitation. Research done at the Tele-Health and Neuroscience Institute, Oklahoma City, USA recently com-

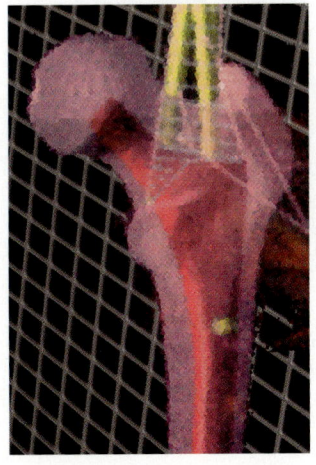

Fig. 60 The pre-planned proposed track of reaming by the use of an intraoperative robotic arm at the proximal femur in total hip replacement

pared conventional vs. virtual reality training platforms for CTS (carpal tunnel syndrome) postoperative rehabilitation.

This paper presents a proof-of-concept pilot clinical trial in which the Rutgers Masters II haptic glove (Figs. 61, 62) was tested on five patients 2 weeks post-hand surgery. Participants trained for 13 sessions, 30 min per session, three sessions per week, and had no conventional outpatient therapy. Computerized measures of performance showed group effects in hand mechanical energy (1,200% for the virtual ball squeezing and DigiKey exercises and 600% for the power putty exercise). Improvement in their hand function was also observed (a 38% reduction in virtual pegboard errors, and 70% fewer virtual hand ball errors). Clinical strength measures showed increases in grip (by up to 150%) and key pinch (up to 46%) strength in 3 of the participants, while 2 had decreased strength following the study. However, all 5 participants improved the tip pinch strength of their affected hand (between 20 and

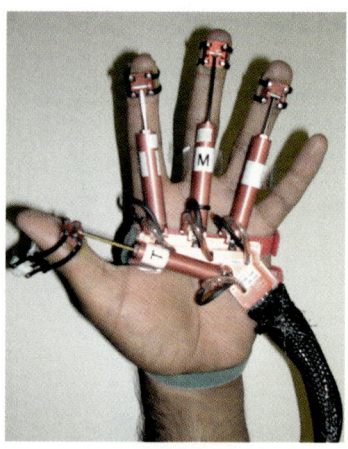 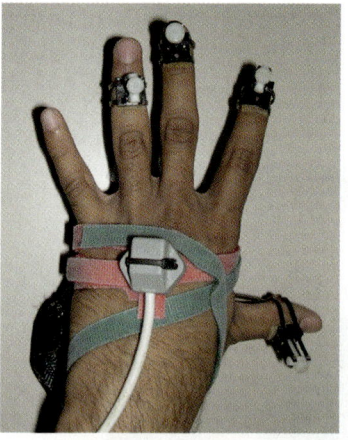

Fig. 61 The Rutgers Master II haptic glove used in hand rehabilitation (e.g., after carpal tunnel syndrome release), front view shows sensorized exoskeleton. © Rutgers University CAIP Center. Reprinted with permission

Fig. 62 The Rutgers Master II haptic glove used in hand rehabilitation, back view shows 3D tracker attachment. © Rutgers University CAIP Center. Reprinted with permission

267%). When asked whether they would recommend the virtual reality exercises to others, 4 participants agreed very strongly and 1 agreed strongly that they would. [Technical note]: The current study is one of the latest studies to confirm that given good graphics and haptic feedback – in this case using the Rutgers Master II haptic glove developed at Rutgers University at New Jersey equipped with haptic feedback capabilities and initially developed as part of a NASA project – the results of such training are promising. The fact that those who experienced the VR platform mention that they will recommend it to others most probably testifies to a good level of immersion in the said VR platform designed for hand rehabilitation.

Use of Virtual Reality in Non-operative Orthopedic Rehabilitation

Example 1: Pain Management

Introduction
It is well known that psychologists use virtual reality to treat phobias through simulations that gradually have patients face feared situations under controlled circumstances. Patients develop control over the fear-inducing stimuli and overcome their fears. In a similar fashion, when physical methods of pain reduction are insufficient, immersion in virtual reality can help patients with long-term pain by taking their mind off the pain

Role of Virtual Reality to Control Pain in the Burns Patient
- Burn injuries and their treatment (such as post-burn limb mobilization exercise and wound care) are considered to be among the most painful a person can endure, especially in young children and adolescent age groups (see Case 41).
- Recently, pain-related brain activity was found to be reduced during immersive virtual reality, confirmed via the use of functional MRI, a new armamentarium in the study of pain.

Literature Support from Research Performed at Washington University Burns Care Unit

A recent piece of research performed at the University of Washington Burns Care Unit by Hoffman and Patterson at the Human Interface Technology Laboratory recruited a group of young burns patients, with a mean age of 22 years and with an average of 24% of the total body surface area burned, were subjected to immersive virtual reality treatment (Hoffman et al., International Journal of Human-Computer Interaction, 2001). It was found that VR continues to reduce pain (via distraction) with repeated use. The name of the game is SnowWorld, a virtual environment created with Creator™ modeling software and VEGATM development software from www.MultiGen.com.

SnowWorld depicts an icy 3D virtual canyon with a river and waterfalls. Patients shoot snowballs at snowmen and igloos by aiming with their gaze and pressing the spacebar on a keyboard. The snowballs exploded with animations and 3D sound effects on impact. Each patient participated in the VR condition, during which they performed active assisted physical therapy exercises.

Meanwhile, the occupational therapist held the patient's injured limb (e.g., arm), and the therapist moved the patient's limb through a predetermined sequence of ranging exercises, while the patient was in virtual reality (e.g., raising the patient's arm as if they were asking a question, or crossing the injured arm across the patient's chest). With adequate VR distraction, an initially painful therapy session can be turned into a more enjoyable useful session.

Conclusion: Pain ratings were statistically lower when patients were in VR, and the magnitude of VR pain reduction did not diminish with repeated use of VR.

[Technical Note]: A Silicon Graphics Octane MXE with Octane Channel Option (www.sgi.com) was coupled with a V8 VR helmet (www.virtualresearch.com) to create an immersive, 3D, interactive, computer-simulated environment. Eyepieces on the helmet were circular and had 60° diagonal field-of-view per eye. A Polhemus Fastrak™ motion sensing system (www.Polhemus.com) with 6df sensors was used to measure the position of the user's head.

[Author's Note]: Recapitulate in the companion volume to this book published by the author that distraction or any intervention that makes the brain neglect the painful sensation is useful.

Virtual reality can function as a strong non-pharmacologic pain reduction technique for burn patients during physical therapy. The results of the study from the University of Washington suggest that virtual reality does not diminish in analgesic effectiveness with three or more uses. Virtual reality may also have analgesic potential for other painful procedures or pain populations.

In contrast to what would be expected if VR was operating solely through a placebo mechanism, in the present study the effectiveness of VR analgesia did *not* diminish with repeated VR treatments and all 7 patients showed VR analgesia.

Practical Case Illustration (Case 40):
Virtual Reality in Burns Care for a Child

History and Examination
A 14-year-old girl called Jane sustained second-degree burns to her face, upper chest, and both hands after trying to reach for a pot of hot porridge 6 weeks ago. She has been under the combined care of the rehabilitation team and plastic surgical team of your hospital. Her mother notices that she is increasingly withdrawn and refuses to come out of her room, let alone go back to the hospital for physiotherapy. When alone, Jane spends most of her time either watching television or surfing the internet.

In a recent multi-disciplinary meeting, the feedback of the clinical psychologist of your rehabilitation team detected a very depressed mood while she talked to Jane, with low self-esteem, and fear of going to places with many people like the supermarket or shopping mall. She disliked the idea of going back to the hospital wards, for it tended to bring back memories of arterial lines, multiple injections, etc., during the time when she was initially admitted to the acute ward. In view of the depressed mood as well as the imminent intent to forsake further rehabilitation, the team members decided to resort to the use of virtual reality platforms to help in this scenario. What is your opinion and how would you proceed from here?

Discussion

Introduction

In this instance, you have decided to employ the "pain distraction system" from a company known as Fifth Dimension Technology (www.5dt. com).

5DT Virtual Reality Pain Distraction System

The objective of the 5DT Virtual Reality Pain Distraction System (VR-PDS) is to distract the attention of patients who undergo painful procedures from the pain associated with the procedure. VRPDS is aimed at painful procedures (e.g., wound-dressing for burns victims) where anesthesia is not a viable option.

The patient wears a head-mounted display (HMD) during the procedure. The HMD fully immerses the patient in the distraction game. The HMD also serves to isolate the patient from the procedure, since the patient cannot see the procedure being performed. The patient controls the distraction game with either a game pad or a joystick.

The distraction games were designed to provide a rich sensory experience. Fast-moving, colorful, and interesting imagery provide visual stimulation. A variety of background sounds and music provide aural stimulation. Force-feedback by the game controls provides tactile stimulation. The games are interactive and require serious concentration. The games also offer a challenge to the players. There are various game levels to keep the patients interested.

There are also games that cater for the very young aged between 3 and 8 years by the name "Jolly Jumpin' Jellies." The game features a fantasy virtual world with "Jolly Jumpin' Jellies," a play park, a rainbow, boat rides, birds, butterflies and the main character "Gotcha." The patient controls "Gotcha" to catch the jellies. There are seven jumping jellies that must be caught in the shortest possible time. Each progressive game level provides faster jellies that are more difficult to catch.

For the older child and adults of all ages, patients may try the game "Street Luge." It is essentially a downhill racing on a big skateboard, with the game player lying on his/her back on the skateboard (Fig. 63). The game features a fast-moving reality-based virtual world. Whereas the premise of the "Jollie Jumpin' Jellies" game was to provide a very stimulating world with cute bubbly characters for pain distraction, the premise of "Street Luge" is a game that requires a lot of concentration and that challenges the game player to try for a better time again and again. Each progressive game level features a higher gravity value, resulting in increasing downhill speeds for the Luge.

Current Case Scenario

Jane agreed to participate in the pain distraction program. During immersion in the virtual world, you arranged community nurses to go to Jane's home to change the dressings on her limb wounds, and perform physiotherapy exercises for Jane. Slowly, Jane adapted to the new program, showed improvement in her functional status, and become less socially isolated and withdrawn than before.

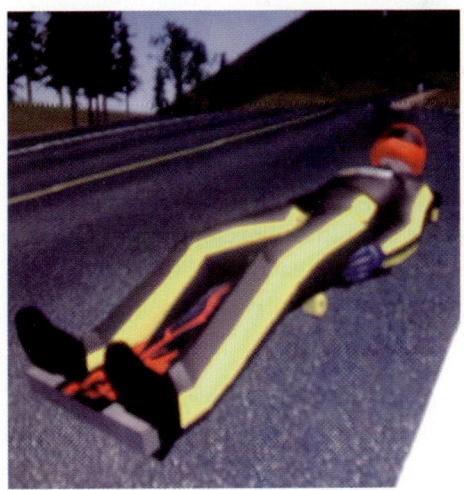

Fig. 63 A scene from the fantasy world of the 5DT pain distraction system (courtesy of 5DT.com)

Learning Point

- When clinicians talk about "pain", what crosses their mind usually includes questions like: "Is it nociceptive or neuropathic?", "Is there centralization?", and "Is there associated psychosocial disturbance?" and so on.
- However, the above and other basic science research studies reveal there is another a new dimension that is often not talked about, which is one that we may use in future to tackle chronic pain. The new dimension to circumventing pain is to make the brain not pay attention to the pain, i.e., pain is still perceived, but there can be ways to tackle the brain pathways so that the brain itself ignores the perception. While this can sometimes be achieved by stereotactic surgery, simpler, non-invasive methods include the use of pain distraction systems in a virtual reality platform designed in such a way as to allow whole-hearted "immersion" of the individual and make him forget the painful sensation.

Example 2:
Ankle Rehabilitation

Introduction
Virtual rehabilitation represents the combination of computers, special interfaces, and simulation exercises used to train patients in an engaging and motivating way (Burdea et al., IEEE Trans Rehabil Eng, 2000). Rehabilitation of different orthopedic conditions can either be clinic-based or home-based. In addition, as an ensuing section will show, it can also be done via long distances in a format known as tele-rehabilitation, done through a virtual reality platform.

Role of Virtual Reality in Ankle Rehabilitation in the Clinic
One such virtual reality platform was developed at the Center of Advanced Information Processing (CAIP) at Rutgers, the state university

of New Jersey. The Rutgers Ankle Rehabilitation Interface features a haptic interface equipped with a robotic device known as a Dual Stewart Platform Mobility Simulator and was presented at the International Conference of Rehabilitation Robotics (ICORR) at Chicago in 2005. It allows patients to interact with motivating virtual environments as they exercise. The device allows movement in all three of the ankle's degrees of freedom through patients' full range of motion. It is capable of supplying both low and high forces in all directions, permitting a large variety of exercises. Because it interfaces with a computer as a virtual reality haptic interface, the system acts as an input/output device to and from virtual environments (Figs. 64, 65). For example, patients can steer a virtual airplane with their feet, feeling resistive forces increase with speed. While patients exercise, the system collects force and position data in all of the ankle's six degrees of freedom.

Literature Support from Research at a Center for Advanced Information Processing at Rutgers University at New Jersey

The results of the above Rutgers Ankle Rehabilitation Interface have been published already. The program has evolved from an initial clinic-based program, currently to be designed for home use as well as internet-based remote monitoring by therapists or tele-rehabilitation-based

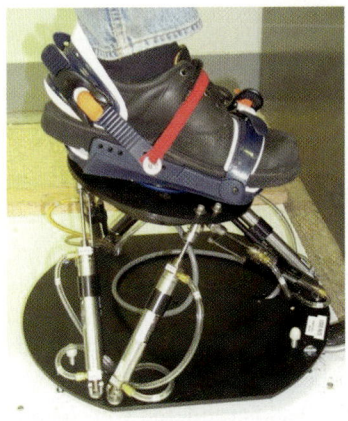

Fig. 64 The Rutgers ankle rehabilitation system: The pneumatic robot. © Rutgers University CAIP Center. Reprinted with permission

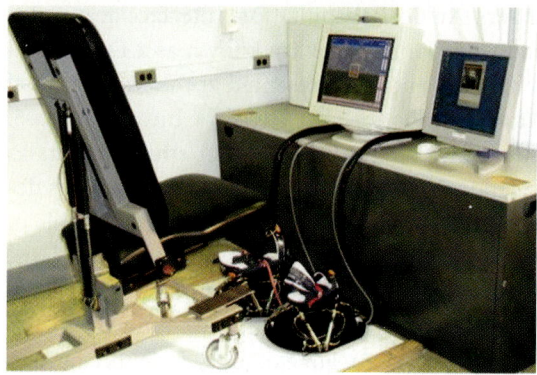

Fig. 65 Rehabilitation station including virtual reality simulation display and remote therapist communication console. © Rutgers University CAIP Center. Reprinted with permission

VR platform capabilities. The Rutgers Ankle VR platform is designed for patients who need ankle and knee rehabilitation. It has been applied in the rehabilitation of patients with orthopedic injuries (ankle sprain) and in stroke patients.

Literature support of orthopedic ankle sprain injuries with the Rutgers Ankle VR platform is found in Girone et al., Proceedings of Medicine Meets Virtual Reality 2000. Its application in rehabilitation after stroke is found in Deutsch et al., Presence (MIT Press) Vol. 10(4), in August 2001.

Example 3:
Training the Patient in the Use of Assistive Technology

Practical Case Illustration (Case 41):
Virtual Wheelchair Training

History and Examination
Paul is a 17-year-old triplegic cerebral palsy patient. He used to be able to walk with a rollator as the right lower limb retained reasonable power, with a GMFCS level of 3. Ever since the adolescent growth spurt, his spastic muscles have not seemed able to keep pace with his longitudinal growth in height and body weight and Paul is rendered wheelchair-

bound. Paul attends a special school, but was teased by two classmates as being rather clumsy and dependent as Paul's mother needed to wheel him around because of Paul's left upper limb weakness. Paul is determined to improve his level of dependence and maneuverability by having a discussion with a rehabilitation specialist like you. How would you proceed?

Discussion

You prescribed Paul an electric wheelchair after discussing with the bioengineer and members of your multi-disciplinary team when Paul attended your seating clinic. However, in view of the fact that Paul had triplegia, you also wish to check for his truncal and neck control, as well as checking in detail the agility of the right upper limb and hand and hand-eye coordination. In the final stage, before Paul was allowed to use the electric wheel-chair to shuttle around the busy streets, you referred Paul for virtual reality training (Figs. 66, 67) to ensure he has the adequate skills and responses to maneuver the electric wheelchair.

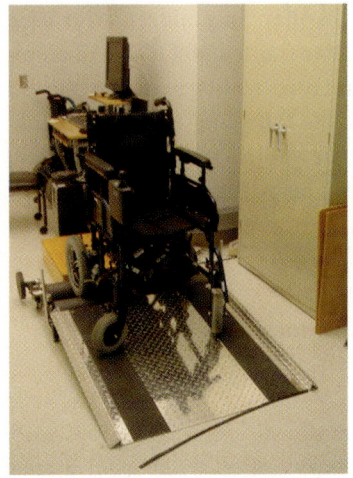

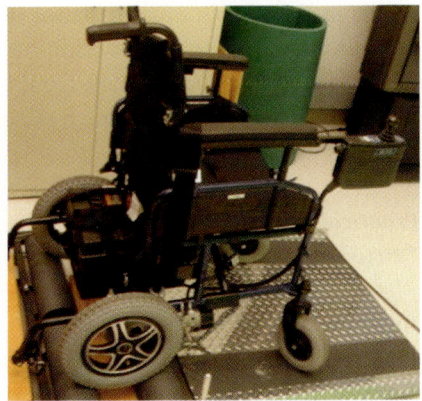

Fig. 66 Wheelchair with built-in software for virtual reality training

Fig. 67 Another view of the wheelchair together with the nearby large monitor screen

Learning Point

- The adolescent growth spurt is a frequent precipitating factor for deterioration of ambulation status of cerebral palsy children as the longitudinal growth of spastic muscle frequently lags behind longitudinal bony growth.
- Not infrequently, some adolescents find it depressing to accept the altered ambulation. An electric wheelchair is a useful assistive device on this score, but special caution should be exercised in those children with upper limb weakness. In situations such as these, virtual reality training will be an advantage before the patient can safely ambulate in the community.

Example 4:
Improving Quality of Life Through the Use of Music

Introduction

As most occupational therapists will agree, the main occupation of young, particularly preschool, children, is play. In children who love music, but who have a disability such as after trauma, to be able to enjoy music in the setting of a virtual or augmented reality platform can be appealing for the patient. In addition, as the following case example illustrates, one added advantage from the viewpoint of the rehabilitation specialist is that the VR platform indirectly helps encourage the child to use the upper extremity.

Practical Case Illustration (Case 42):
"Virtual Music" in Upper Extremity Rehabilitation

History and Examination

Jane is a 9-year-old right-handed girl in a local grammar school who suffered a right upper brachial plexus injury after a fall from a tree branch, who was treated by your orthopedic unit initially with neurotization and later with Steindler flexorplasty and derotational osteotomy of the shoulder.

Despite treatment by dedicated physiotherapists and occupational therapists, Jane was noted to use her right upper extremity less and less in daily living. Prior to the injury, she enjoyed very much listening to music and playing the piano. In a multi-disciplinary meeting with the therapists, in the presence of her mother, the team decided to let Jane re-use her right upper extremity by the use of a VR platform. Do you think that a VR platform can encourage Jane to use her right upper extremity again?

Discussion

In the present case scenario, the use of a virtual environment is used to help achieve our patient carry out her main occupation, i.e., play, or more specifically, playing of music. The concomitant expected benefit from this is enhanced use of the affected extremity.

The virtual music instrument (VMI) illustrated in Figs. 68 and 69 works by a "teacher"/therapist controlling the master notebook computer and the patient seated in front of the big screen (Fig. 70). When-

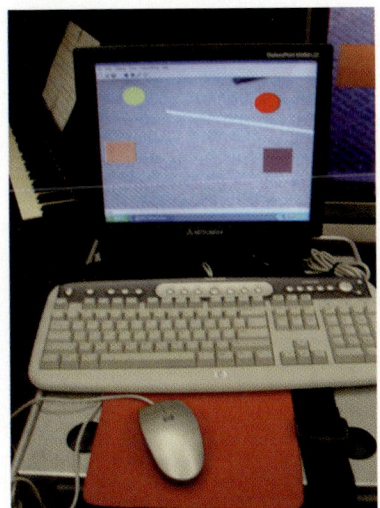

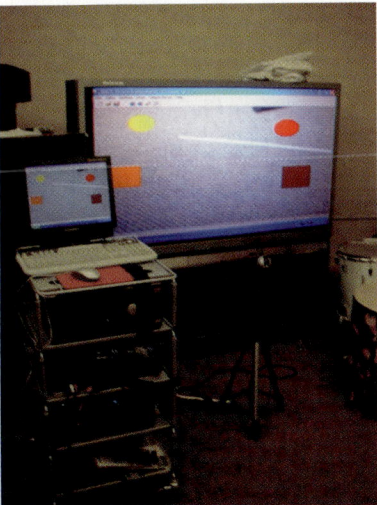

Fig. 68 Computer used by the teacher of the Virtual Musical Instrument

Fig. 69 Large monitor screen used to project the image to the patient

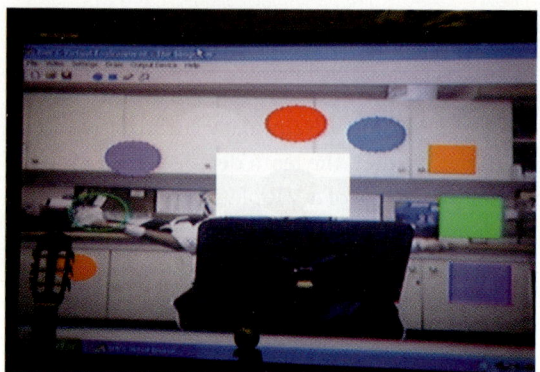

Fig. 70 Note the change in color of the circle to transparent when the patient's hand is positioned to the music note she desires

ever she uses her arm to reach for the colored circles (e.g., the yellow or red circles as illustrated in the figures), she will hear a certain musical note. Hence, by a suitable array of circles arranged by the computer on the monitor screen, the child will be able to play her own beloved song and music.

In the present case scenario, Jane resumed active use of the arm after a 2-month course of VMI, despite residual weakness in right shoulder abduction and external rotation, and resumed active participation in the therapist's protocol of rehabilitation of her right upper extremity.

The idea of virtual music stems from the desire to allow physically disabled children who have difficulty in assessing traditional music instruments to play music. The technology was pioneered at the PRISM laboratory at the Bloorview Kids Rehabilitation Institute in Toronto, Canada.

The program developed at Bloorview Kids Rehab is known as VMI or Virtual Music Instrument and was designed by Tom Chau and coworkers. VMI was presented in the USA at the RESNA meeting, and at the AAATE meeting in France (Chau et al., 2006). A similar program was extended to include the rehabilitation of the elderly with dementia (www.lifecare.org.au/).

The potential advantages of the use of VMI include encouragement of the physically disabled patient (can be children or the elderly) to use their upper extremity, stress reduction, enhancement of self esteem, participation in music enjoyment, and playing via a virtual reality platform.

Learning Point

■ The advantages of virtual music are manifold. Besides helping to fulfill the performance and enjoyment of music in disabled children with upper extremity weakness, the actual layout encourages the child to use the weakened extremity. This is especially the case in a child with unilateral upper extremity weakness (e.g., residual weakness after brachial plexus injury), for the longer a child disregards the weakened extremity, the less likely it is that he/she will eventually use the extremity. This may make the effort of the physiotherapists and occupational therapists futile.

■ Besides being extremely useful in the rehabilitation of childhood disability, the more recent report of its potential use in the rehabilitation of dementia patients by aiding and enhancing the visuo-construction ability of dementia patients (Tarnanas, Stud Health Technol Inform, 2000) as well as the elderly with upper limb weakness and disability appears promising.

Tele-rehabilitation

Tele-rehabilitation is the provision of rehabilitation services at a distance, by a therapist at a remote location. Traditionally, tele-rehabilitation has been administered through video conferencing and video phones, without the use of virtual reality.

Tele-rehabilitation is a relatively new tool in orthopedic rehabilitation. The idea behind it is that the patient trains with the help of a therapist at a remote distance, and the patient feedback parameters are relayed to the therapist. The therapist analyzes and transfers new training instructions back to the patient. One example of such a computer-aided training platform is the Universal Training Assistant, adapted for the training of postoperative total joint replacement patients by Eisermann et al. from Austria.

More recently, virtual reality has been integrated into tele-rehabilitation, representing a relatively new addition to this field. Tele-rehabilitation aided by virtual reality can be clinic-based or home-based. In a clinic-based tele-rehabilitation environment, an assistant therapist at a remote or rural clinic is coached by an expert therapist in a tertiary care (or university) setting. For home-based tele-rehabilitation, the patient trains at home while being monitored by a remote therapist at the clinic. An example of tele-rehabilitation in orthopedic rehabilitation is the training of ankle rehabilitation at Rutgers University and is done across the east and west coast of the USA.

Literature Support of the Use of Tele-rehabilitation with a VR Platform in Hand Rehabilitation

One such VR platform can be found at the Center for Advanced Information Processing (CAIP) at Rutgers University, headed by Dr Michael Pazzani, who is located at the Computing Research and Education Wing of Rutgers University at New Jersey.

One of the on-going projects at CAIP is known as the "Multi-Modal Tele-Collaboration Laboratory Project." The Multi-modal laboratory involves a system that allows two participants to work collaboratively on a specific task with one participant (the novice) working in the real world, being guided by another participant (the expert) using virtual overlays to the experience of the novice. In hospital patients before discharge, this can be done by the therapist guiding the patient prior to discharge to rural areas far away from the hospital.

A PC-based orthopedic rehabilitation system was developed for use at home, while allowing remote monitoring from the clinic. The home rehabilitation station has a Pentium II PC with graphics accelerator, a Polhemus tracker, and a multipurpose haptic control interface. This novel interface is used to sample a patient's hand positions and to provide resistive forces using the Rutgers Master II (RMII) glove. A library of virtual rehabilitation routines was developed using WorldToolKit software. At the present time, it consists of three physical therapy exercises (DigiKey, ball, and power putty) and two functional rehabilitation exercises (peg board and ball game). These virtual reality exercises allow automatic and transparent patient data collection into an Oracle database. A remote Pentium II PC is connected to the home-based PC over the internet and an additional video conferencing connection. The remote computer runs an Oracle server to maintain the patient database, monitor progress, and change the exercise level of difficulty. This allows for patient progress monitoring and repeat evaluations over time. The tele-rehabilitation system is in clinical trials at Stanford Medical School, with progress being monitored from Rutgers University. Other haptic interfaces currently under development at the above institutions include devices for elbow and knee rehabilitation connected to the same system.

Combined Use of Tele-rehabilitation and Virtual Reality in Postoperative Orthopedic Conditions

Practical Case Illustration (Case 43) on Hand Rehabilitation

History and Examination

Joanne is a 12-year-old school girl who lives in a rural district far away from any nearby hospital. Six weeks ago, she cut her left index finger helping her mother in the kitchen, and completely divided the flexor tendons in Zone II area with active venous bleeding. She was sent to the nearest county hospital where she received surgical repair and inpatient rehabilitation. However, the wound became infected and she had another operation done. Postoperatively, Joanne felt depressed and reluctant to undergo different physical and occupational therapy sessions.

Upon discharge from the hospital, Joanne has residual stiffness in her injured finger. The multi-disciplinary rehabilitation team is worried about residual disability, particularly since it was the index finger that was injured. Joanne's mother further commented that since Joanne has to return to her school and they live very far away, it is not practical for

Joanne to come back for therapy sessions. After much discussion, the multidisciplinary team finally arranged tele-rehabilitation for Joanne. The clinical psychologist of the team in fact found that despite the fact that Joanne was depressed and reluctant to undergo therapy, she very much enjoys playing computer games and games consoles.

Luckily, Joanne's elder brother has a quite advanced computer at home as he is studying for an on-line university degree; thus, the multi-disciplinary team decided to provide further training through a virtual reality platform (Figs. 71–73). As for supervision of the therapy, this will be done via a web-based camera as well as by video-conferencing.

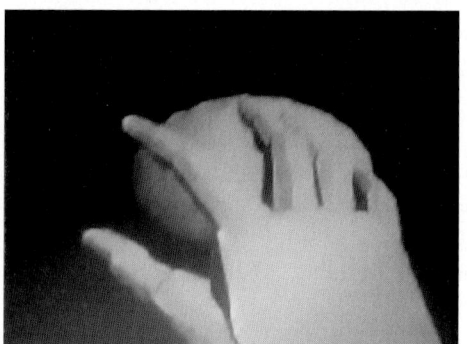

Fig. 71 Virtual hand reaching for a ball

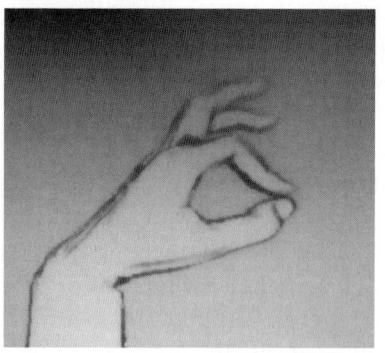

Fig. 72 Virtual training of a fine pinch grip

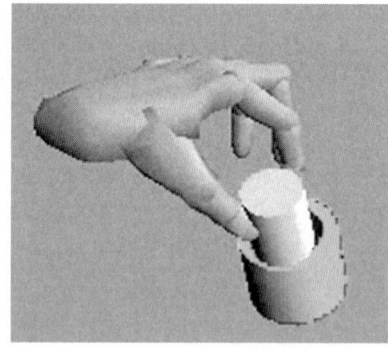

Fig. 73 Virtual training in picking up fine objects

Discussion

The idea of the importance of tele-rehabilitation first occurred to the author with the knowledge that some operations done in children with disabilities by orthopedic surgeons in some developing countries do not want to come back for rehabilitation because of cost concerns and the long distance between their home and the major hospitals. Tele-rehabilitation can help reach out to these difficult scenarios, as long as their home has a telephone line for data transfer.

Present Case Scenario

Training hand function in virtual environments involves special interfaces such as 3D trackers (for wrist movement), or sensing gloves that measure finger joint positions in real time, thus enabling the sensing of the different gestures of the hand. One such interface at this time is the haptic glove, which can apply computer-controlled resisting and/or assisting forces at the finger level.

The VR rehabilitation system used in this study consists of a PC (Pentium III dual processor), a 3D tracker by Polhemus, left- and right-hand haptic gloves by immersion.com with their control box, and a Canon pan-tilt-zoom camera controlled over the internet. The haptic gloves are used to measure in real time the thumb, index, middle, and ring fingertip positions vs. the palm. Custom actuators resist flexion or assist extension to the neutral hand configuration. A remote therapist expert looks at the PTZ camera images through a web browser, communicates with the local therapist over the phone and has access to the patient treatment/history through a web portal. Joanne proved to be an intelligent patient and learned to enjoy the exercises taught by the therapist, including modified exercises recommended by the famous hand surgeon, Palmer.

Learning Point

- There is an increasing number of rehabilitation specialists, including the author, who propose more and more home monitoring and home treatment programs. Examples are given throughout this book like virtual hand rehabilitation, home monitoring by infrared thermometer in diabetes patients with a high risk of ulceration, but concepts of tele-rehabilitation are most important in less affluent countries where patients do not have ready access to rehabilitation resources after, say, surgery. In this connection, the combined use of tele-conferencing and virtual reality will definitely be helpful and welcomed by poor patients living in areas far away from hospitals and clinics.

- Tele-rehabilitation in the present context involving a PC-based orthopedic rehabilitation system was developed for use at home, while allowing remote monitoring from the clinic.

- There are long-reaching consequences for the future as this technology potentially allows patients living in rural areas a chance of continued rehabilitation after surgery at a medical center in the city. This is especially important in a vast country like China in which, despite there being many modern medical centers in major cities, many patients living far away have difficulty in returning to major hospitals for rehabilitation.

- Another good point about the tele-rehabilitation in progress is the potential to monitor the patient's progress at a distance as long as the patient's computing system is connected to the main computer at a designated medical center equipped with VR facilities. Some may argue that VR facilities also involve costs, but this is much less expensive than building a hospital complex and requires comparatively much less time to set up.

Other Clinical Applications of Virtual Reality

Cognitive Rehabilitation

The reader is probably aware of the ever-expanding geriatric hip fracture population, especially in Asia and the Asian-Pacific region, which contains two-thirds of the world's population. Studies performed by the author have shown that as the population ages, the number of the elderly who fall because of the intrinsic factor of falling as opposed to the extrinsic factor (such as tripping over an obstacle, or wet floor) is likely to increase.

As one major aim of rehabilitating hip fracture patients is to try to retain them as community walkers instead of being housebound or sent to nursing homes, *concomitant* cognitive rehabilitation can be an useful tool in this respect in managing the so-called "oldest old," a common term used by geriatricians. In many parts of the world, including the author's home country, there is an increasing number of elderly people using the computer and surfing the internet. This trend certainly opens a door with room for cognitive rehabilitation of the elderly suffering particularly from fragility fractures of the lower extremity that can potentially jeopardize their mobility. As for the actual VR platform, one example is the more recent report of the potential use of virtual music in the rehabilitation of dementia patients by aiding and enhancing the visuo-construction ability of the dementia patients (Tarnanas, Stud Health Technol Inform, 2000). Other VR platforms conducive to cognitive training are under investigation in some VR centers in Washington.

Stress Reduction by the Use of VR Biofeedback

At the Biofeedback Center at Reno, Nevada, USA, Dr Green and colleagues are using virtual reality to manage anxiety disorders, for stress relaxation, pain management, and to inculcate a sense of self-help and self-improvement, which the orthopods can introduce to their patients with chronic disability (Fig. 74). Those interested can visit Dr Green's website at www.stresslesslife.com/vrbiofeedback.htm.

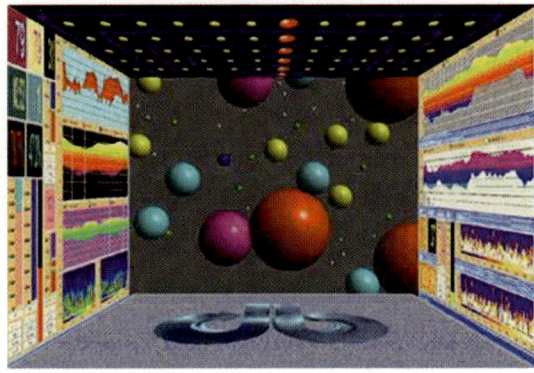

Fig. 74 A scene from a VR platform used by Dr Green. Courtesy of Dr Green, Nevada, USA

As an Aid in Biopsychosocial Interventions in the Future

In Washington, USA, there is on-going research in the Research Center for Virtual Environment and Behavior. Here, researchers are interested in the experience of social presence as well as task performance within collaborative virtual environments. Researchers are utilizing virtual reality simulations in which people interact in real-time within a collaborative virtual environment. Specifically, they seek to:

- Learn more about the behaviors that occur during collaboration
- Explore the idea of transforming social interaction by selectively augmenting and decrementing these behaviors in order to provide the participants with novel tools during interaction

Thus, immersive virtual environments may, in future, allow for conversational strategies that are somehow not possible in face-to-face interactions or video-conferencing. Researchers are examining the effect of implementing these novel strategies, and testing their influence on conversation in terms of task performance, learning, and persuasion. It is the author's view that these said strategies are of potential help in trying to help some injured workers return to work whose reason for not returning is mainly psychosocial in nature.

Virtual Tomography

Virtual tomography puts together several CT or MRI scans of body organs and systems with simulated kinesthetic interfaces.

Given the aid of virtual visual and kinesthetic systems, surgical training robots simulate the look, feel, and response of real patients for physicians who are learning how to diagnose illness and provide treatments. Sophisticated kinesthetic systems allow physicians-in-training to move their hands along with the recorded hand movement of an expert to learn the best technique.

Cost Concern

Currently, high-resolution virtual reality play is not economically feasible on a large-scale, distributed basis. However, this will probably change with the continuing advances in computing power and the development of lower-cost VR hardware. In fact, provision of VR platforms for patients in rural areas of a huge country where many resources are centralized in big cities is much cheaper than building new hospitals in the different rural areas, which requires lots of money and time on the part of the local health authorities.

The Future

In the author's opinion, there are three areas worthy of development as far as the clinical uses of VR platforms are concerned.

Group Therapy in the Future Via a VR Platform

With multi-participant online virtual reality, in which groups of people participating can come into contact virtually, participants can gain the benefits of group exercise without the costs of tangible travel, and represents a cost-effective way of training.

Generating the Ultimate 3D Effects

The formation of micro-lens and arrays of micro-scale mirrors with transparent polymers is opening up an innovative generation of 3D imaging. Arrays of micro-scale lenses constructed of polymeric materials can be directed to converge using compression or expansion with piezo-electric currents. The interaction of holo-technology laser images with micro-scale lens or arrays of micro-scale mirrors can lead to genuinely three-dimensional moving images.

VR and Robotics

Virtual reality can also help surgeons to discern the boundaries of diseased tissue and remove it from healthy tissue nearby. Medibots guided by virtual reality enable micro-surgery on a micro-scale and with greater accuracy than is possible with traditional surgical operations. Thus, the large-scale motion of a physician by control panel devices is translated down to the micro-scale movements of the robotic components within the patient.

Summary of References for Section II

General References

1. Web source: www.caip.rutgers.edu (Rutger's Ankle and Virtual Hand platforms)
2. Web source: www.5dt.com/products/pvrpds.html (Pain Distraction Software)
3. Grigor C, Burdea G (1996) Force and Touch Feedback for Virtual Reality. Wiley-Interscience
4. Sherman WR, Craig A. Understanding Virtual Reality: Interface, Application, and Design (The Morgan Kaufmann series of Computer Graphics)

Journal References

1. Hoffman HG, Patterson, et al. (2001) The effectiveness of Virtual Reality pain control with multiple treatments of longer durations: A case study. International Journal of Human-Computer Interaction, 13:1–12
2. Carlin AS, Hoffman HG, et al. (1997) Virtual reality and tactile augmentation in the treatment of spider phobia: A case study. Behaviour Research and Therapy, 35:153–158
3. Hoffman HG, Holander A, et al. (1998) Physically touching and tasting virtual objects enhances the realism of virtual experiences. Virtual Reality: Research, Development and Application, 3:226–234
4. Székely, Satava (1999) Virtual reality in medicine. BMJ, 319:1305
5. Chau T, Schwellnus H, et al. (2006) Augmented environments for paediatric rehabilitation, technology and disability. 18(4):167–171
6. Schwellnus H, Chau T, et al. (2002) Using Movement to Music Technology to Facilitate Play in Children with Special Needs. Occupational Therapy Now, 4(6):11–13
7. Knox R, Chau T, et al. (2005) Movement-to-music: Designing and implementing a virtual music instrument for young people with disabilities, International Journal of Community Music, 2(1)

8. Tarnanas I (2000) A virtual environment for the assessment and the rehabilitation of the visuo-constructional ability in dementia patients. Stud Health Technol Inform, 70:341–3

9. Popescu VG, et al. (2000) A virtual-reality-based telerehabilitation system with force feedback, IEEE Trans Inf Technol Biomed, 4(1):45–51

10. Burdea G, Popescu V, et al. (2000) Virtual reality-based orthopedic telerehabilitation. IEEE Trans Rehabil Eng, 8(3):430–2

11. Haik J, Tessone A, et al. (2006) The use of video capture virtual reality in burn rehabilitation: The possibilities. J Burn Care Res, 27(2):195–197

12. Dennerlein JT, Diao E, et al. (1999) In vivo finger flexor tendon force while tapping on a keyswitch. J Orthop Res, 17(2):178–84

13. Heuser A, et al. (2007) Telerehabilitation using the Rutgers Master II glove following carpal tunnel release surgery: proof-of-concept. IEEE Trans Neural Syst Rehabil Eng, 15(1):43–9

14. Monkman GJ, Boese H, et al. (2003) Technologies for haptic systems in tele-medicine. Stud Health Technol Inform, 97:83–93

Subject Index